Healing from Cancer
A Call to Freedom

Antonia G. Milo, Ph.D.

Disclaimer

The contents of this book are not intended to be taken as a
substitute for medical consultation and treatment, nor as supportive of
avoiding or going without medical consultation and treatment.

ISBN 0-9653664-2-1
Library of Congress
Catalog Card No. 98-094872

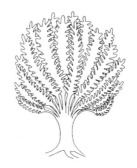

Balanced Way®
P.O. Box 785
Fernandina Beach, FL 32035
1.800.523.2403
http://www.balancedway.net

Balanced Way® is committed
to using recycled or tree-free paper.

Printed in the United States of America

Cover and book design by Frank A. James,
Hamilton Press, Fernandina Beach, FL.

Contents

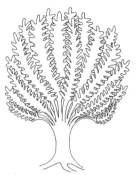

Introduction

This booklet is the product of my experience with "cancer." It also includes what I have learned from the experiences of friends who were sick, and from related books and articles.

My experience with "cancer" began in August of 1980 when I suddenly noticed a big lump in my breast. On December 1, my gynecologist measured it. It was about 2 and 1/2 inches by 1 and 1/4 inches. A mammogram taken on Christmas Eve of 1980 revealed a one-centimeter mass with "sunburst" extension into the surrounding tissue, "a probable carcinoma.." I began my healing meditations and soon after, began eating completely vegetarian food.

Two surgeons to whom I was referred recommended mastectomies. This scared me. A wonderful surgeon kindly carried out a diagnostic excision biopsy, on my terms: under local anesthetic, on March 20th, 1981. He removed two lumps which had tentacles (he showed them to me). One lump was nearly round at 3/4 inch, the other narrow: 1/4 inch wide and over ½ inch long, without their tentacles. The diagnosis was infiltrating lobular carcinoma of the breast, with perineural invasion.

After the surgery, my occasional pains became more frequent and intense. On April 1, I consulted a prominent authority on breast cancer who told me he thought that my "cancer" had spread to the lymph nodes on the opposite side of my neck and to my colon. On May 2, I attended a "Diet and Cancer" public seminar given in Boston by the Kushi Institute and I began to eat a piscovegan (very occasionally fish, plus plant food) diet tailored to my health needs. I was already following a clean lifestyle without knowing it.

My lifestyle was close to "macrobiotic" to start with. That is, I wore natural fabrics, used no chemicals in medication or cosmetics, and very few in household cleaning; I exercised vigorously nearly every day by walking up and down little mountains or by swimming a half mile; I ate little meat and drank coffee but no soft drinks and rarely a glass of wine, all of this by inclination. I did not smoke, either. Where I lived was not far from the Vernon, Vermont nuclear power plant, and a woman had died of cancer in the farmhouse in which I lived. Because I was so fit, it was quite a shock to be diagnosed with cancer; but this is a shock for anyone. Still, it caused me to wonder: what was I doing wrong?

The way I ate to heal myself was and is very effective. I can see from my own experience how strongly what we eat can influence our moods. Therefore much, but not all! of this book is about food. Together with breathing and resisting gravity, eating is our most intimate physical act of communion with our world. It is the only one in which we may exercise a significant amount of choice.

After careful consideration, I refused, as I had before, the mastectomy, the chemotherapy and radiation that were recommended at two leading medical centers of the Northeast.

My experience with "cancer" did not end one and one half years later when scans of my lungs, bones, uterus and ovaries revealed no evidence of it. That event was perhaps the end of what I call the 'active healing' phase of my disease. The healing way of eating that I began a few months after my diagnosis of breast cancer continues to this day, as does my wonderful lifestyle which includes simple but active living, involvement with nature, and time for myself, just to be peaceful or to meditate. I have long ceased to worry about a recurrence because I know why I got cancer, and I know how to move it out.

What I call the 'passive healing phase' of my cancer overlapped with the active phase of healing and continued for seven years, after which I felt fully restored to health.

I noted that for seven years, I had occasional breast pains. The pains usually came after experiencing unpleasant emotion: a combination of disappointment, shock and despair. To a lesser extent, and sometimes not at all, the pains were associated with eating in a way that could be threatening to my health.

These pains awoke in me the same fear and anxiety that I had lived with when I had "cancer." "It's back!" I thought. Until those pains, and the feelings that came with them! left for good, I consider that I still had the sickness called "cancer."

After those seven years had passed, I called myself "cured."

The second or third year after my diagnosis, it came to my attention in a roundabout way that I had not only physical but mental/emotional work to do in order to improve myself. This realization moved me to take six meditation courses in Shelburne, Massachusetts, at a center dedicated to the practice of *vipassana* meditation,[1] a Buddhist spiritual discipline which does not conflict with the beliefs and practices of Islam, Christianity, or Judaism. These courses are given on a donation basis.

The Buddhist courses were supplemented by courses in "Creative Living," taught by Dr. Alex Tannous at the Uni

---

[1] as taught by S.N. Goenka in the tradition of Sayagyi Uba Khin. Sayagyi Uba Kin taught this form of meditation as it had originally been taught by Gautama Buddha, the teaching having maintained its purity through the centuries in Burma.

versity of Southern Maine School of Nursing.[2] These courses involved hypnotic self regression and traveling back through time to correct mistaken beliefs which had resulted from past events. (They were 35 dollars/ c.e.u.)

A joint workshop given by Alex and Chuck Spezzano, Ph.D., extensively applied the "healing of memories"[3] to ancestral traumas. I learned that the experience of our ancestors lives in the descendants who carry it, although rarely for more than five generations, in their "genetic memory."[4]

The work of Rupert Sheldrake, which is becoming accepted by the scientific community, recognizes that an invisible (to us) "morphogenetic field" is a template for our physical form.[5] The morphogenetic field is one aspect of the "etheric body" or "energy body" which is the focus of acupuncture, homeopathy, radionics and many other healing methods.

Much is being made today about genetic mutation and cancer, whether inherited (5-10% of cases), induced by pollution or by "chance."[6] In the future, people may find that the genetic mutation which accompanies cancer may itself be the response to a disturbed "morphogenetic field" which has been distorted by unhealed emotions and resulting mistaken beliefs of long standing.

The occurrence of a mutation during the course of a lifetime shows us that the DNA of our single cells or of populations of cells can change. If, through introspection and meditation, we heal the emotional patterns and correct the mistaken beliefs which adversely affect our morphogenetic field,[7] and if we change our exposure to injury from the

---

[2]Alex Tannous, Dr. Div., 1983, 1984:c.e.u. courses, University of Southern Maine School of Nursing.
[3]Ruth Carter Stapleton, "The Experience of Inner Healing," World Books, 1977.
[4]The work of Rupert Sheldrake, Ph.D. ("A New Science of Life: the Hypothesis of Morphic Resonance," Tarcher 1982) supports the concept of 'genetic memory.'
[5]Rupert Sheldrake, Op. cit.
[6]Tim Friend, Whys, hows of breast cancer start with genes, USA Today, March 10, 1998, p.5D.

external factors which promote mutations that are associated with cancer, why wouldn't future populations of our cells appear in a healthy form? Two principles in biology suggest that they might. One is *homeostasis*, the self correcting mechanism that is almost synonymous with life. The second is an aspect of homeostasis. It is: *healing is a property of living tissue.*

By acting in such a way as to change our "morphogenetic field," can we not become masters of form and of our own mutations? The question is: how to do it.

*　*　*

At the same time I realized that clearing myself of emotional and mental bad habits is the work of a lifetime, I began to offer support to persons with cancer who were referred to me as a result of my success. But I would not call it 'success'. I would call it my 'blessing'.

My healing from "cancer" was the result of the grace that allowed me to place myself increasingly in harmony with Nature (the Great Healer) and myself, through my attitude and through the way I lived.

I did not attempt to make war on my "cancer" but rather to understand it, to make peace with Nature, and to turn darkness into light within myself.

Antonia G. Milo

---

[7]Stylianos Atteshlis, On the Etheric Double (for Psycho-therapists), *General Lecture*, Feb. 7, 1991, *audio cassette*, Nicosia.

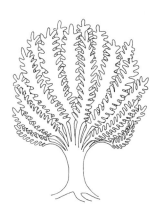

Chapter One
Definitions

Before sharing some things I learned, it is important to offer some definitions which for me have changed as a result of my experience with cancer. I shall begin with a definition of "cancer."

Cancer
What is "cancer"?

"Cancer" is not a "thing" but a degenerative process which is not immune to nature's laws. It is known under one name in the West, but what we Westerners call 'cancer,' in the Orient is several different diseases. From the standpoint of Oriental Medicine, the Western term 'cancer' is a catch-all for imbalances of different kinds which affect us physically, emotionally and mentally simultaneously.

Too, in the West, the causes of cancer are not understood. Certain conditions, environmental and physical and even mental and emotional have been observed in association with the occurrence of "cancer," and certain substances and conditions produce "cancer" in laboratory animals, but how this widely varying and variable disease occurs is still a mystery. The likelihood of getting "it" can only be defined in terms of probabilities, and once one has "it," no one can say what the outcome will be for any given individual. Such a prediction is based only on statistics.

In response to questions, physicians may and do make predictions, sometimes less tactfully than a psychic hotline might do. When asked, they may say such things as: "You have six months to live," or "only chemotherapy could save you now." Most physicians positively do not know when they, or anyone else, are going to leave the physical plane because every person is different. Every person is very possibly going to prove a prediction wrong. So many have.

We all can be tortured by uncertainty. When we ask our physician "how much time" we have, we may be asking the wrong person. If we are a physician who is asked such a question, do we want to deliver a negative opinion to a sick and therefore a highly suggestible and frightened person? If we are such a person, do we have to believe it?

If the positions of doctor and patient were reversed, no doctor would allow himself or herself to make predictions. The worst thing about predictions is that a person with cancer is likely to believe them, then to imagine them. We all know where human nature goes from there: to acting out one's imagination. What we do with our imagination is vital, especially when we are sick and therefore vulnerable to suggestion.

We know two things about "cancer."
1) It has many causes.
2) It also has many cures.

Cure
What is a "cure"? In order to answer this question, we need to contrast "cure" with "healing." "Cures" are objective. They can be or are recognized by someone else. "Healings" are subjective and are recognized by the individual concerned.

Cures and Healings may, but do not always, coincide.

A person may feel and be healed but not cured. But can a person be cured and not healed?

Healing restores wholeness, a person's feeling of wholeness. To feel *whole* is to feel in touch with Life beyond the existence of our mere personality. This may be desired more urgently by a sick person than is physical existence. It sometimes takes a disease such as "cancer" to restore or to bring that feeling of wholeness about.

A life threatening illness gives a person space for healing and change which one might possibly find otherwise only by taking holy orders, and less favorably, in solitary confinement.

Holistic medicine seeks healing and is patient.

Holistic medicine
What is holistic medicine?

Holistic medicine may be contrasted with conventional Western, "allopathic" medicine. Western medicine is called 'allopathic' because it treats sickness and disease as something foreign to the individual. At the same time, it treats the body as a closed system. This is a paradox. Holistic or alternative medicine sees the body as an open system which includes the environment and all of nature as well as one's own feelings, thoughts and activities. By treating the symptoms of disease, Western medicine tries to eradicate it. We may add that Western medicine is truly a product of our age.

Oriental medicine, based on an ancient system which describes the whole of Creation, treats disease as the manifestation of an imbalance between the two primary attributes, Yang and Yin, each of which is lethal when imbalanced. The relationship between these attributes is further expressed in the balance between the five energies that pervade the physical world and all things in it.

Technological miracles of Western medicine have resulted from collaboration of the best and most highly trained scientific intellects. We marvel at the fact that it is possible to reconnect to the body a limb which has been severed in an accident, or that a valve of the heart may be repaired or replaced—even an entire organ—and that it is now possible to clone animals and people. But, although the incidence of cancer is decreasing, the "War on Cancer" admittedly continues to be lost. Could it be because making war is counterproductive? In our judicial system, mediation is now being encouraged in order to avoid battle.

What about viewing cancer not as an enemy but as an ally or a teacher which leads us deeper into the meaning of our existence? We may view cancer in this way if we believe that there is more to us than our physical body, a belief which is an active part of holistic medicine.

Whomever I asked felt as I did: that their cancer or AIDS was the best thing that had ever happened to him or her, whatever the outcome of his or her illness might be. This attitude is widespread in those who persist in healing themselves naturally. It is also found in at least some women with breast cancer, whatever therapy they may follow.

A valued friend, who has suffered great damage due to cancer in her family, objected to my calling my cancer a "friend." "After all, it *is* trying to kill you," she wrote. But that would make it an enemy, and I do not see cancer as the enemy. If the cancer cells have conscious intent, it is surely not to kill us but, as cells in our body, to obey the dictates of a greater order, whether those dictates were set by different kinds of pollution, by sudden stress, by unfortunate experiences or by a combination of factors.

Michio Kushi says that our culture's hostility to disease results from attributing it to an external source rather than to our lifestyle and cultural behavior.[9] Our lifestyle can protect us from many kinds of pollution which have caused

---

[8]Antonia G. Milo, lecture presented at *12th Int.Conf. On the Study of Shamanism and Alt. Modes of Healing*, 1995a, *audio cassette*.

14

sickness and death to so many creatures and beings.

Could it be that the materialism of our age has limitations? It has removed our focus from the spiritual, not only within Nature, but within ourselves. Respect for our bodies and for our selves is necessary for health. The humanity of so-called 'primitive' societies and of ages past long recognized that we exist simultaneously in many dimensions, not only in this physical world. Think about it. When you are daydreaming, you are existing and active in a dimension that is not physical. And what you do in your imagination and with your emotions affects your conditions in the physical world.[10] [11]

1. Holistic medicine is so called because its practitioners believe that disease affects the (w)hole person: body, feelings/mind and spirit. Good illustrations of holistic medicine are the healing centers of ancient Greece, which were derived in turn from the mysteries of ancient Egypt, and current shamanic healing practices. At the ancient, holy places dedicated to healing, people would speak with healing priests and spend the night in search of a healing dream. People would be set on the path to healing by prayer, physical treatments and by their own dreams.

A holistic practitioner is likely to view the physical body as a road map of mental and emotional conditions.[12] For instance, asthma may be associated with a situation in which a person feels that he or she is being smothered by some aspect of his or her existence. Similarly, a craving for sweets and even diabetes may express an unrequited longing for greater sweetness in one's life. Hypnotic regression has been used to heal physical conditions having an origin

[9]Michio Kushi with Edward Esko, "The Macrobiotic Approach to Cancer". 1991, Avery Publishing Group, Garden City, New York, pp.18-21.
[10]Milo, *unpublished manuscript.*
[11]O. Carl Simonton, Stephanie Matthews-Simonton and James L. Creighton, 1978: Getting Well Again: a Step By Step, Self Help Guide To Overcoming Cancer For Patients and Their Families," Bantam, New York.

in events from even one's sometimes far distant past.[13]

2. Unlike allopathic, or conventional medicine, holistic medicine addresses the cause rather than the symptoms of a disease. Holistic practitioners do not focus particularly on physical symptoms but on the condition of the whole body. They understand that the body's condition will affect a person's mind and feelings and that a person's mind and feelings will affect the condition of his or her body.

3. Holistic medicine understands and relies on a mystery of Nature and the body, of which Western medicine, in cases of chronic illness, seems not to take advantage. It is this: Life itself is healing.

Holistic medicine is based on and works with what we may have learned in a biology class: the principle of *homeostasis.* Homeostasis is the innate, self regulating mechanism that causes our body temperature to remain almost the same in winter and summer, indoors and outdoors, clothed and unclothed.[14] It miraculously causes our wounds to close, colds to pass away, broken limbs to heal. Furthermore, this principle is part of us and never leaves us, no matter how sick we are. From it, we gain the understanding that:

4. A living organism or human being functions as a whole. If you help any part of yourself, you help the whole person.

---

[12]Christiane Northrup, M.D. "Women's Bodies, Women's Wisdom," 1994, Ballantine, addresses this truth extensively in working with female disorders.

[13]Brian Weiss, M.D. "Through Time Into Healing," Simon and Schuster, 1992. Chapter 4: *Healing the Body by Healing the Mind*, pp. 56-76.

[14]Within a limited range of outside temperatures.

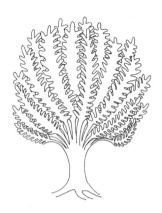

Chapter Two
A Different Medicine

Time and "cancer"

When I was diagnosed with breast cancer, and did not yet know which course of treatment I would follow, my father was a greater help to me than he could ever know. He said to me: "Take your time. You know what is good for you. Take your time."[15] What an idea... I did take my time! Some months later, at the medical center where I was getting a second opinion about radiation and chemotherapy, a nurse there was very helpful to me also. Her mother, she said, had been in and out of the hospital with cancer for years. This nurse confided to me that "the patients who take their time to choose a treatment until they find one they really believe in, do the best."

Persons with cancer are usually rushed into surgery, radiation or chemotherapy before they have time to think about it. This is because physicians are concerned about doubling time. That is, a tumor does not grow in a linear way: two cells, then three, four, five cells, etc. Instead, the

---

[15]At one point when I was quite anxious to take action, my physician reminded me that my tumors had taken between five and eight years to reach the size they did, so a few months more or less would not make much difference. But cancers vary in their growth rate.

more it grows, the more it grows: two cells, four, eight, six-teen, thirty-two cells, etc. That is why physicians feel that time is of the essence when confronted with a diagnosis of "cancer." To a physician who is focused on the tumor(s) which is one of the symptoms of "cancer," time is an enemy.

To a holistically inclined person, doubling time may not mean so much because having a little bit of "cancer" is like being "a little bit pregnant." But with cancer one is dealing with a process which can be reversed.

"Cancer" and time

Frightened and anxious though I was, I did not rush into a treatment without taking my time. I waited until I had confidence in it, that it was the best thing that I could do for myself. But in order to take my time, I had to manage my considerable anxiety. In fact, when I had cancer, managing my anxiety took more time than anything else. The spiritual, psychological and physical means with which I successfully managed my anxiety are described in my pamphlet: *A Double Axe: Cancer and the Mind.*[16] We shall discuss some of them at the end of this book.

Taking one's time to select a treatment or treatments one believes in means that one is taking responsibility in getting well. It means making decisions oneself instead of letting someone else make them for you. Many physicians are now realizing that the patient should be, and is, included as part of the treatment team.

Furthermore, we are not all the same. Some of us would prefer to grit our teeth, bite the bullet and blindly go forward, trusting in our inner strength, in God, in Life, and do not want to participate in any decision making of a medical nature. We are in this case taking responsibility for our-selves on another level, the level of faith.

We may also share a deep trust and understanding

---

[16]1996, Balanced Way, Fernandina Beach, Florida.

with our physician who may even be a family friend of many years.

Taking immediate action after a diagnosis of cancer has the very great advantage of not giving us time to imagine the worst, time to agonize, time to worry. Our worry may be deferred as we wait to see how well the treatment has worked.

A friend of mine did not leave the hospital following her diagnosis of breast cancer. She was kept in overnight and had a radical mastectomy the next morning. But her physician was a trusted family friend who had delivered her daughters many years before. He assured her that it was not her breasts that made her the human being and woman she is. He said of her breast: "This is only a piece of meat. It has nothing to do with you or your body."

The friend cited above, whose husband had died of cancer leaving her with two daughters to support, eventually simply knew within herself that everything was going to be all right.

A "Cancer personality"?

Interest in the relationship of cancer to personality and behavior has revived. There is an increasing, recent body of clinical studies on this subject, a review of which is beyond the scope of this book. The work I mention is what was most relevant to my experience and which, I feel, may most inform a person with cancer or AIDS. Exceptions which we shall discuss later are studies of *self transcendence*: that is, going beyond oneself to love, serve and help others. According to my own experience, this may be the best tonic for any illness.

Excluded from the medical literature is the work of Dr. Geerd Hamer of Germany. He has found that with a precondition of being exposed to double bind situa

---

[17]Dr. Med. Ryke Geerd Hamer, "Krebs, der Krankheit das Seele," Verlag Amicidi Dirk, 1987, Koln: Gesellschaft Med. Schriften.

tions (heads, you win; tails, I lose) in childhood, a person may develop "cancer" within five to eight years after a severe unresolved emotional conflict or injury and within one to two months after a second such emotional conflict has occurred.[17] One might say that cancer which occurs in association with such conditions has a spiritual cause as a person becomes disheartened and loses faith in his or her existence. All of this certainly was true for me.

Some women with breast cancer are claiming that breast cancer is an expression of a disturbed relationship with one's father. I would say that in our society, in which such a high value is placed upon competition and winning, the qualities of daughters may indeed be cherished by their fathers, but fathers may not know how to express this in a nonsexual, supportive way. But the real causes of disturbance, even in familial relationships, are one's own negative feelings and mistaken beliefs.

It took me years to see the members of my family of origin and myself as the people we were or are. My main obstacle to reaching this point of peace and balance were in fact not my parents, but my own desires and beliefs. I was projecting onto my family the beliefs I had absorbed from the society at large and wanting things to be different. I interpreted the fact that my father had spent little time with me as indicating that I was not worth it, when many demands were being made of him.

Since the Industrial Revolution, our home life has been shaped by the need for shift work. Fathers became absent with a separate life from that of their family in our economy and in wartime.

Some parents assume that their children are extensions of themselves or part of a family "group soul" and do not show their love. They assume their children know what they are feeling. Some families do not have a tradition of seeing a child's needs or of meeting them, because their own needs were not met. And among some people, fathers hold the mistaken belief that they own their children.

It took having "cancer" for me to open myself enough to learn that people care. My parents certainly loved me, but due to circumstances not of their making, I closed myself to believing it and learned to not care, myself, about my feelings. Having grown up and got on with my life, I continued as an adult in the idea that others do not care what I feel, what I think, what I need. How could they care? Because I never expressed those things to others, and rarely to myself.

An emotional cycle which rings true to me has been identified in connection with "cancer": perceived rejection which is followed by perceived betrayals by persons one trusted, followed in turn by increasing isolation from others.[18] This certainly was my experience and what I have seen of friends I have known who had "cancer."

J. Rodale, the founder of *Prevention* magazine, has written a book which includes comments by physicians from other centuries, titled "Happy People Don't Get Cancer."[19]

Iemoshok and Dreher[20] have assembled a vast array of data which suggest that the denial of one's needs and feelings result in a "cancer personality." To begin to express oneself is a vital ingredient in physical recovery. Particularly valuable, I thought, were Temoshok's citing of the importance for persons with cancer of the "one-second realization." The section "Signposts on the bridge between mind and body"[21] elaborates on this. I recommend the whole book—browse it if you wish, including footnotes at the end.

"Cancer" and space

The pioneer of our age in the study of the feelings of persons having "cancer," Lawrence LeShan, Ph.D., has

---

[18]Conversation with a friend, Sun City, Arizona.

[19]J. Rodale, 1970: "Happy People Rarely Get Cancer," Rodale Press Inc., Emmaus PA.

[20]Lydia Temoshok, Ph.D. and Henry Dreher, "The Type C Connection: the Mind-Body Link to Cancer and Your Health," Plume, 1993.

[21]p. 247 and pp. 266-268: signposts on the bridge between mind and body.

found that having "cancer" offers an opportunity for change in which people find out or identify what they want to do but have not been doing with their life. Discovering and doing what they want to do has been associated with physical improvement and /or with healing in the truest sense, when "death" is accompanied by peace and satisfaction with the fullness of one's existence.[22]

If you think about it, where do we go in our society when we want to make a change? Where can we go, if we are caught up in the demands of a marriage, a family, a job, or simply in the routine of our existence? We need to go into a different space within our selves, and "cancer" offers us this opportunity.

If our need for change were not so profound, we might not find our life at risk. By developing a life threatening condition, we change not only physically but psychologically and spiritually. Physically sick, the outer world fades while the richness of our inner life (if we are not taking drugs to relieve our anxiety and pain) increases as our perceptions change.[23] [24]

It is well known by now that our state of mind affects our health, just as it is well known that sickness and/or other physical stress affects a person's state of mind. In fact, it is now being suggested that emotions affect our genetic material. Is it too far fetched to think of certain genes as transducers for positive and negative emotional energy?

It is also possible that poor eating habits may lead to a vicious circle in which physical sickness and accompanying emotional malaise are the outcome.

[22]Lawrence LeShan, "Cancer as a Turning Point," Plume, 1990.
[23]Milo, manuscript in preparation.
[24]Milo, 1996.

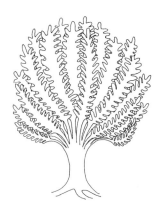

Chapter Three
Other Challenges to Health

In school I was taught that once people reach a certain age, they are likely to live much longer. People I know who have lived to be old, that is, well past eighty, are vigorous and mentally alert so I now consider that old age begins at eighty. Such individuals have caused me to consider the environment in which they were raised and its effect on their mind and body. They grew to adulthood before the United States began to produce one ton of chemical wastes per person each year.[25]

The National Cancer Institute a few years ago revised upwards their estimate of the incidence of "cancer" in the population of the United States by the year two thousand from one third to one half the population! Why?

An extensive overview of agents that contribute to carcinogens can be found in *Women's Health 2*.[26] A brief review here of some of the ways in which our environment differs now from what it was in "the good old days" may show us something.

---

[25]Kushi, 1991, p.23.
[26]Burton Goldberg, "Alternative Guide to Women's Health 2," 1998, Future Medicine Publishing, Tiburon California: pp. 62-82.

Cancer and pollution

The association between "cancer" and the pollution is fairly straightforward, especially where the development of all our children is concerned. I refer you to the newsletter of organizations such as *Public Citizen, Mothers and Others*,[27] and back issues of newspapers.

Everyone is so pleased that the overall incidence of cancer is decreasing. But childhood cancer rates are climbing approximately 1% each year and cancer is the common fatal form of childhood disease.[28] Pollution that is associated with the incidence of cancer comes from many facets of our physical environment.

First, there are the household toxins that we live with and may sleep with every night. They include not just radon gas, especially in certain geographical areas, but PCBs (polyvinylchlorides) which are released into the air as vinyl products gradually deteriorate over time and formaldehyde which is part of foam insulation (it is also used in embalming). Ingested through the lungs in breathing, these substances tax our liver and kidneys. Carolyn P. Gorman's original list of more common toxic household products and non-toxic alternatives to them is well worth reading[29] as is the work of Dr.Clark,[30] *Toxics A to Z: A Guide to Everyday Pollution Hazards*[31] and the editors of *every issue* of *The Green Guide*.

Dr. Ernest Sternglass, former Professor *Emeritus* of Radiology specializing in radiological physics at the University of Pittsburgh Medical School, and Ralph Graeub, a chemical engineer who is an expert on the dangers of

---

[27]*The Green Guide,* 40 West 20th St., New York NY 10011-4311, 888/ECO-INFO.

[28]*The Green Guide, June 1,1998, (54/55).*

[29]1993, "Less Toxic Living," sixth edition, Environmental Health Center, 8345 Walnut Hill Lane, Dallas Texas 75231.

[30]Hulda Regehr Clark, Ph.D.,N.D., "The Cure For All Cancers," 1993, ProMotion Publishing, San Diego.

[31]Harte et al.,U.C. Press, 1991.

atomic energy, have presented data concerning not only the association of background nuclear irradiation and the incidence of cancer in children[32] but damage to the environment as well, due to the Petkau Effect, which is the genetic damage inflicted by steady, long-term exposure to even minute amounts of background radiation (of which there is plenty).[33]

The occurrence of cancer in the United States between 1974 and 1991 increased, especially the incidence of leukemia among young children,[34] while it is on public record that the sperm count in the United States and northern Europe has been dropping since 1954.[35] Could the drop in sperm count and the increase in childhood leukemia be, in part, to the results of unpublicized but evidently widespread (more widespread than we may know) underground nuclear testing?

We do not know the long-term effects on Earth life of the explosions at Hiroshima and Nagasaki. It has been said that the world will never again be the same after Chernobyl.

Radiation from the Chernobyl explosion has traveled around the entire earth, although documentation of some of its effects have occurred nearer to the blast. For example, the growth of trees in the Black Forest in Germany has decreased by fifty-four *per cent.* Think of that! This is only one of the effects on our environment, and presumably on us also, that has been noted as a result of that explosion.[36]

Electrical fields can be another carcinogenic influ

---

[32]Ernest Sternglass, 1981, "Secret Fallout" with *Introduction* by George Wald, McGraw-Hill paperback edition, an expanded version of "Low-Level Radiation" first published in 1972 by Ballantine Books.

[33]Ralph Graeub, 1992: "The Petkau Effect" with *Introduction* by Dr. Ernest Sternglass., Four Walls Eight Windows, New York. Translated from the German by Phil Hill. Revised English edition of 1990: "Der Petkau-Effekt," Zytglogge Verlag, Bern.

[34]Gurney J.G., Davis S., Severson R.K., Fang J.Y., Ross J.A., Robison LL., Trends in cancer incidence among children in the U.S. Cancer, Aug. 1,1996 78(3): 532-541.

[35]Michael D. Lemonick, What' s wrong with our sperm? *Time Magazine,* March 18, 1996: 78-89.

[36]Graeub.

ence. Paul Brodeur's three articles in *The New Yorker* Magazine in 1989 first brought this matter to public attention and was followed by two books on the subject.[37] [38]

Land near electrical substations, power lines and large transformers is usually cheaper. Brodeur described the high incidence of cancer in elementary-school children whose school was adjacent to a California utility company's electric substation. An Internet National Medical Library (http://www.nlm.nih.gov) survey of abstracts of articles published in 1995, '96 and '97 under the search heading "cancer, electromagnetic fields," overall indicates that there can be a significant increase in the incidence of cancer with prolonged exposure to strong electromagnetic fields. The difficulty with such studies seems to lie in quantifying the data.

Then there are "cancer houses," It has been noticed and studied in Germany that the people who live or work in certain buildings tend to get cancer. The cause has been attributed to either a viral cause of cancer, which has not been ascertained, or to "noxious influences" at the location. These "noxious influences," which can be identified and transmuted by the oriental science of *feng shuei,* have been studied and even modified by dowsers here and abroad.[39] [40]

Dowsing is also known as "water witching," but this is not witchery. Dowsing is the manifestation, as a physical response, of changes in the earth's energy, which occur when veins of water or other materials running beneath the earth intersect there. If yours is an animist view of the cosmos, meaning you believe that everything has consciousness, then the Earth's energy field itself, as well as the perturbations in it, are expressions of different levels of

[37]Paul Brodeur, "Currents of Death," Simon and Schuster, 1989.

[38]_____, "The Great Powerline Cover-Up," Little, Brown and Co. 1993.

[39]Christopher Bird, Progress in Getting the Medical Profession to Focus on the Study of Geopathic Zones and their Effect on Health, *The American Dowser,* 24 (4): 6-13. November 1985.

[40]Christopher Stone, First Geopathic Congress on Geopathic Stress in Cyprus, 1997, in *The American Dowser* 38 (1):32, Winter, 1998.

intelligence.

Pesticides have been implicated heavily in cancer. DDT, so common in the thirties, forties, and fifties,has been banned. But many of the pesticides in use today contribute especially to breast cancers by chemically resembling female hormones or substances that promote excessive production of the female hormones implicated in some breast cancers.

And there is air pollution. The air in much of the United States may or may not be substantially cleaner than it is in those areas exposed to heavy automobile and industrial pollution. For example, the smog from Washington, Baltimore, Wilmington, Philadelphia, New York, New Haven, Providence and Boston rolls in an increasing wave up the northeastern seaboard after business hours until it reaches the Acadia National Forest on the Northern Maine seacoast at about two o'clock in the morning, where it has been killing the trees. The pines in Acadia National Forest have been dying.[41] Also, the haze from Los Angeles is visible not only over the Grand Canyon but over most of northern Arizona.

Autopsies reveal that the lungs of a person who has lived in the country, at death are a clear and uniform pink. The lungs of a city dweller, by contrast, are grey due to being heavily flecked with black pollution.

Air pollution enters our lungs where it is trapped, particularly if we smoke, reducing the efficiency of our lungs and thereby promoting an acidic condition, or, entering the bloodstream, causing further work for our liver and kidneys.

When singing with other people, someone who is ninety-two can hold a note longer than I can! Why? He grew up in a clean rural environment; I grew up in a dirty urban one and, on top of childhood exposure to smog and

---

[41]On June 24 of 1998, new smog limits set last summer had been exceeded by at least thirty states and the District of Columbia. The American Lung Association said that violations had occurred "in all regions, including every Eastern State except Vermont and Rhode Island," Levels of smog raising alarm, *USA Today,* Wed. June 24, 1998, p.5d.

DDT, I used to smoke. Perhaps smoking is associated with cancer because decreased lung capacity results in systemic acidosis. That is to say, the fluid plasma surrounding our cells is not well oxygenated.

Pollution is especially serious for the young ones whose bodies are developing and therefore much more sensitive to pollutants of all kinds. We can expect infertility and the incidence of all kinds of diseases to rise. The incidence of leukemia in children has risen globally already.

The Rev. Hanna Kroeger has called attention to the introduction of viruses of animal origin through inoculation programs, some of which are retroviruses which may remain dormant in the body for years.[42] Without citing any sources, she suggests that viruses and fungi, acting alone or in combination with each other, with metals and with parasites, can cause cancerous tumors and many other diseases.

Last, but most definitely not least, of factors associated with an increased incidence of cancer is diet.

We ingest the alcohols and benzenes that promote the establishment of parasites in our internal organs in many of our processed foods and drinks.[43]

The food we eat can cause cancer. "Half of a lifetime's consumption of carcinogens from food is eaten by age five."[44]

According to the late Dr. Virginia Livingston, persons with cancer respond to a change in diet coupled with injections made from an extract of their tumors. Dr. Livingstone felt that cancer is caused by a virus and that this virus is closely akin to, if not the same as, the notorious Rous sarcoma virus in chickens.[45]

Whether we have cancer or not, it is possible that

[42]Rev. Hanna Kroeger, Ms. D. "Free your body of tumors and cysts," 1997, Hanna Kroeger Publications.
[43]Clark.
[44]Harvey Karp, M.D., quoted in *The Green Guide,* June 1, 1998, (54/55), p.2.
[45]Virginia Livingston, M.D., "The Conquest of Cancer," Livingston Foundation Medical Center, San Diego.

detoxifying ourselves and making the condition of our blood more alkaline rather than acidic is beneficial in building up our resistance to colds, flus and other infectious agents.[46] Can we detoxify our blood and tissues and build up our resistance to infections without damaging our bodies further?

[46]Herman Aihara, "Acid and Alkaline," George Ohsawa Macrobiotic Foundation, 1971 (first edition) Oroville, California.

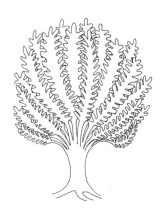

Chapter Four

By Bread Alone?

It has been said that "cancer" is a disease of malnutrition. This could be so for at least two reasons. The colon may be impacted, preventing the full absorption of nutrients, on the one hand, and on the other, the food we ingest may itself be polluted in several ways and also have little food value.

Yes, there are toxins in much that we eat in the form of preservatives, artificial flavor enhancers and artificial coloring, but the food we take in may be poor in value, such as refined white flour and soft drinks. People rely on refined white flour products and soft drinks a lot, especially if they are uninformed about nutrition or have little money for food. But we have a single bad habit which is characteristic of the Western diet. It is: eating high on the food chain.

What does it mean to "eat high on the food chain"? It means eating animals or fish or fowl that have eaten other animals, fish or fowl. When you eat an animal, fish or fowl that only eats fruits, nuts, vegetables and possible insects,

---

[47]Noboru Muramoto, Chapter 2, *Plagues and Epidemics,* pp. 27-44, and Chapter 3, *The Meat Eater's Body,* pp. 45- 60 in"Natural Immunity: Insights on Diet and AIDS," 1988. George Ohsawa Macrobiotic Foundation, Oroville.

such as free-ranging chickens or game birds do, one is still eating high on the food chain which, historically, has been associated with death from plagues.[47] To eat low on the food chain is to eat plant foods.

Eating high on the food chain, first of all, exposes us to a wider variety of environmental toxins because chemicals in the plants that animals, fish or fowl eat are stored in the creature's fat.

Do you remember how people were avoiding tuna fish because of the high concentration of mercury that was being found? This was due to the tuna eating smaller fish who ate still smaller fish who carried in their bodies the mercury absorbed by the plankton, krill and seaweeds growing in areas of pollution of sea water due to industrial wastes.

Dairy products are extremely susceptible to radiation because milk is fatty. Any radioactive fallout goes directly into the milk of nursing cattle and other herbivores. Nearly all of Europe threw away its stock of milk and cheese immediately, and for some time after, the Chernobyl disaster.

The flesh of animals also may harbor substantial pollution that their growers routinely place there: for example, antibiotics in chickens who are heavily laced with them from the moment they hatch, and growth hormones in meat.

In the 'eighties it was reported that in Puerto Rico, where the hormonal content of the meat was unregulated, children: from the ages of two to nine had developed adult female breasts—among other things. Could this be in part why meat-eating members of Western industrialized societies are having fertility problems?

Could the decrease in sperm count noted over the last fifty years be associated with a decreasing average age

---

[48]According to Marcia E. Herman-Giddens, Ph.D., writing in *Pediatrics*, April, 1997, cited in , *The Green Guide*, June 1, 1998 (issues 54-55) p. 4., in a study of 17,000 girls, 48% of black girls and 15 % of white girls had begun to show signs of puberty between the ages of eight and nine. What are the reasons for this, and why the racial differences?

of puberty[48] in American girls? Could both these changes be at least in part because of the sex hormones, indistinguishable from those of human origin, which are "implanted in the ears of more than 90% of commercially raised feedlot cattle"?[49] Our medical standards for what is a healthy amount of exposure to hormones and chemicals is not based on childrens' tolerances, but on the tolerances of adult men.

Could the increase in diseases which are resistant to antibiotics be related to eating poultry that is routinely fed antibiotics? Thanks to Mad Cow disease and Oprah Winfrey, it is now widely known that much of what domestic animals eat is the meal made from the flesh, bones, innards and skins of other animals. This applies to poultry as well. Chickens, as well as family pets, are fed chick meal: the squashed, minced bodies of male chicks in pellet form.

The last liability associated with eating high on the food chain that we will mention here is that this type of food is mainly protein. Flesh is protein. What is wrong with eating more protein than our bodies need? I shall briefly summarize some of the information which has been widely available for some time.

A diet high in protein is a diet which is low in roughage. According to Dr. Neal Barnard, Americans take in only about one half the amount of fiber they need because of eating animal products and plant foods which are refined such as baked goods and baked snacks.[50]

The *diverticula* are the little pouches that are distributed the length of the colon, in which the final part of the digestive process takes place. With a sedentary life and the prolonged consumption of a large proportion of animal products, the *diverticula* of the colon may become impacted and cannot get cleaned out, particularly if you are not taking

[49] S.S. Epstein, The Chemical Jungle: Today's Beef Industry. *Int. J. Health Serv.* 1990, 20 (2): 277-280.
[50] 1993: "Food For Life: How the New Four Food Groups Can Save Your Life," Crown, New York, p. 96. Originally published by Harmony Books, 1993, New York.

the time to chew your food properly. The fruits of an impacted colon are decreased absorption of nutrients, diverticulitis and possibly even a perforated colon, or cancer.

Many civilizations have understood the importance of colonic hygiene. There is, for example, a yoga exercise through which one can learn to flush and cleanse one's colon regularly. The ancient Egyptians also carried out a practice to cleanse their colon as have many other peoples.

A diet high in protein is also likely to be a diet high in fat. People who eat chicken and forgo red meat to protect their cardiovascular system from the effects of "bad" (LDL) cholesterol are not aware that fat is also distributed in the meat and that the meat of chicken contains as much cholesterol as beef does.

Is there such a thing as consuming too much protein? Certainly there is. Americans have tended to eat a lot of protein, particularly since 1916 when the Department of Agriculture came out with five basic food groups, one of which was sweets, another of which was fats, and a third of which was animal products including dairy products, eggs and fish. WWII food shortages led to a revision in which mainly of note was the optional substitution of legumes, beans and nuts for meat by persons with a low income.[51] Thereby, eating meat became a status preference, as was eating white instead of whole-grain bread. As the habit of eating animal products spread through populations with a traditionally low income, mortality due to cancer has increased in them as well.

What about our precious kidneys? A National Medical Library Internet survey of the past two years under the heading: *dietary protein, kidney function*, and related articles, reveals that in people, dogs, rats, mice, and even in little lambs, a high protein diet results in hyperplasia (exces

---

[51]Physicians Committee for Responsible Medicine, P.O. Box 6322, Washington, D.C. 20015. *PCRM Update*, May-June 1991, p.6.

sive increase in size) of the kidneys. A recent, four-month study of 88 volunteers with healthy kidneys who habitually ate widely differing amounts of protein (thirty-two were vegetarian), found that high protein intake significantly affected their kidney function (assessed by creatinine clearance).[52]

If a low protein diet can improve severe and even reverse early kidney disease,[53] [54] [55] might eating smaller amounts of protein than in the standard "Western diet" conserve and promote kidney health overall? Dr. Barnard says that it would.[56] It is evident that eating too much protein can negatively affect the performance of your kidneys.

The importance of our microcirculation may be underestimated. If one removes toxins from and supplies more nourishment to the extracellular fluids that surround our individual cells, might they not respond? The cells of our body have their own life, too.

Our body is constantly renewing and rebuilding itself. For example, bone is willing to remodel itself in response to pressure; that is why people wear braces. If we change and improve their environment, why might not our organs restore themselves according to the genetic blueprint that is carried within each cell?

It is possible that our genetic blueprints themselves may change. How could some of my breast cells become malignant without having changed their genetic blueprint? It

---

[52]However, the subjects had selected their own diets thereby possibly skewing the results. Still, a highly significant correlation was present. Brandle E., Sieberth H.G., Hautmann R.E. Effect of dietary protein intake on the renal function in healthy subjects. *Eur. J. Clin. Nutr.*, Nov. 1996 50(11): 734-740.

[53]S. Klahr, Is there still a role for a diet very low in protein, with or without supplements, in the management of patients wth endstage renal failure? *Curr. Opin. Nephrol. Hypertens.* July, 1996, 5(4):384-387.

[54]Walser, M., Effects of a supplemented very low protein diet in predialysis patients on the serum albumin level, proteinuria, and subsequent survival on dialysis. *Miner. Electrolyte Metab.*1998 24(1): 64-71.

[55]Mackenzie H.S., Brenner B.M. Current strategies for retarding progression of renal disease. *Am. J. Kidney Dis.*, Jan. 1998 31(1): 161-170.

[56]p. 24.

appears to be a property of genes to mutate. Why may mutation not reverse itself to the original form that promoted balanced functioning of cells within their environment? Are the cells in my breasts now behaving normally with abnormal genes? I doubt it! Western medicine has the ponderous view that the *status quo* is forever. The Orient knows that Change is the law. The body is not static but mutable, as are even space and time.

It takes a lot to upset the Balance of Nature. To restore it may take work and self improvement but in a changing, yet orderly Universe, change is not impossible.

Important in eating is our spiritual intent. Healthy individuals vary in their dietary requirements. "For as the Master gave, it is not that which entereth in the body, but that which cometh out which causes sin. It is what one does with the purpose, for all *things* are pure in themselves and for the sustenance of man—body, mind and soul. And remember, these must work together."[57]

The physical and the spiritual are related. Can we cure one without healing the other? We can do both by following Nature, the giver and the given. How? By living simply, remembering that less may be more.

Westerners might consider Abel's sacrifice. Could his sacrifice of flesh imply that he himself was vegetarian, and could Cain, who sacrificed produce, have been a meat-eater? Or did Abel's sacrifice of flesh show greater love because to produce it is so much more costly, in terms of land and plants, and Nature's effort, than is produce?

John Robbins' book, *May All Be Fed: Diet for a New World*[58] is about the high cost of animal food, to our bodies and to crop cultivation worldwide. We should all read it.

While each person seeks his or her own therapy, just as the same physical laws apply to all of us, so do spiritual

---

[57]Anne Read, Carol Ilstrup and Margaret Gammon under the editorship of Hugh Lynn Cayce, "Edgar Cayce on Diet and Health," Warner Books, 1969, p. 29.
[58]1992, William Morrow, New York.

ones: not to be greedy or take more than one's share (what one needs), to respect life, to respect one's body and not put trash in it, even though it has become a way of life to do so.

Since WWII, the USDA guidelines have reduced the "Basic seven" food groups of the Wartime Nutrition Program to Four, as follows: 1. All vegetables, 2. Bread and cereals, 3. Dairy products, 4. Meat, fish, milk and eggs.[59] Naturally, these guidelines had a great influence on American eating habits. Mothers wanted the best they could give their children. Yes, milk and calcium may be good for bones but kale, for example, yields more calcium *per* unit of weight than does milk.

Billions of children have been born and grown to a radiant maturity without consuming any milk product other than that which came from their mother. Dr. Barnard says that the concentration of pesticides is much lower in the breast milk of vegan women: those who eat no flesh nor any animal products.[60] He goes on to point out that not only are pesticide concentrations higher in the breast milk of meat eaters, but that carcinogenic pesticides and industrial chemicals concentrate in the breasts themselves.

I wish everyone could read Chapter Three, "Cancer and Immunity," in Dr. Neil Barnard's book: *Food for Life*, cited above.

Did you know that the excessive consumption of animal protein, which is a "powerful regulator of calcium metabolism" is associated with osteoporosis? [61] [62] John Robbins, in a chapter which is extraordinary - to me, but perhaps not to members of the medical profession - has

---

[59]Physicians Committee for Responsible Medicine.
[60]Neal Barnard, M.D. "Food for Life: How the Four Basic Food Groups Can Save Your Life," Crown, 1994, p. 66.
[61]Barnard, pp.19-20.
[62]See also Kerstetter J.E., Caseria D.M., Mitnick M.E., Ellison A.F., Gay L.F., Liskov T.A., Carpenter T.O. and Insogna K.L. Increased circulating concentrations of parathyroid hormone in healthy young women consuming a protein-restricted diet. *Am. J. Clin. Nutr.* Nov., 1997 66(5): 1188-1196.

pointed out that, contrary to popular belief, the correlation between dietary calcium and loss of bone is weak and perhaps not significant. He has cited medical research which demonstrates that calcium loss is instead correlated with the consumption of animal protein.[63]

If the senior folk, ladies particularly, cut down on eating the animal protein to which they are accustomed, would there be so many tragic instances of broken bones and deformed spines? Evidently not. The deterioration allegedly due to Grandfather Time evidently has more to do with our eating habits.

The health professionals who carried out a study of sixteen healthy young women (all within two years of being twenty-six) found it "unsettling" that the dietary allowance of protein for adults, published by the National Research Council (1989) and recommended by the World Health Organization, is close to the amount of dietary protein which they found to induce calcium loss in the young women.[64]

The message of Robbins' and Barnard's books is repeated in many ways, from many sources: we do not need meat, poultry or dairy products in order to have enough protein, even if we are body builders. Both books also have a wonderful selection of recipes which can be a pleasing and welcome change, especially in hot weather which we now have, thanks to Global Warming. The plant kingdom includes protein—enough to supply our protein needs.

A group of physicians, who are leading us into the third millennium call themselves 'Physicians for Responsible Medicine'. They oppose animal testing, the results of which too often do not apply to human beings. They took a brave step in 1991 by coming out with a replacement for the old Basic Food Groups. They are urging people to eat from the new Four Basic Food Groups. Can you imagine what those might be? They are: 1. Grains, 2. Vegetables, 3. Fruits, 4.

---

[63]Chapter Three: To Grow Up Big and Strong, pp. 57-67.
[64]Kerstetter et al., pp. 1194-1195.

Legumes/beans. But do we follow their suggestions?

Unlike Americans, 70 *per cent.* of whose protein comes from animals in the form of flesh or dairy products, only 70 *per cent.* of the Chinese protein intake is animal protein.[65] Vegetables and especially beans have protein too! But in this country we are accustomed to think of "protein" as "meat," "poultry" or "fish," "milk," "cheese" and "eggs".

[65]T. Colin Campbell, quoted <u>in</u> Study: Meat in diet increases disease risk. *The Boston Herald,* May 9,1990, p. 26. This article is a pre-publication summary of data from the 1990 China-Oxford-Cornell monograph by Chen Junshi *et al.*: "Diet, Lifestyle and Mortality in China," Cornell University Press XVII, 894 pp. Campbell was director of the study of six thousand people.

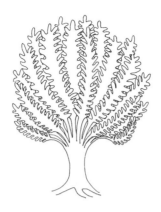

Chapter Five
A Downhill Slide

There is a stage between sickness and health in which one is not sick but one does not feel very well, or look very well, either. Some scientists believe that cancers normally come and go throughout our lifetimes, and that only rarely do they pass the point at which the sickness acquires a progressive momentum to become a downhill slide.

Some results of unhealthy eating

I have mentioned diverticulitis. In connection with eating a low fiber diet, it has been found that "an apple a day keeps the doctor away." Apples coat the colon with a substance that prevents colon cancer.

Another result of a diet which is high in animal foods is fat deposits in and around our vital organs which interfere with their blood supply.

Because animal food stays in our small intestines a long time, it may putrefy there and overwork the kidneys and liver.

When the body is overwhelmed with more animal food and protein than it can handle, tumors may develop.

What is so bad about tumors? They are the body's

attempts to localize toxins in one place. They may be benign but can also be malignant, depending on how toxic the physical environment, our body, has become.

What are tumors made of? I saw mine after they were removed. They are made of what most of our body, and animals' bodies, are made of: protein and fat with very little roughage.

A Canadian physician, Dr. Gaston Naessens, forced to practice outside the United States, through using a special condenser with a dark field microscope, has examined the blood of healthy people and of many people with different stages of cancer. He has found that the sicker a person is, the more concentrated in the blood is the presence of subcellular particles which are neither cells nor viruses. As people recover from their cancer, the number of these particles decreases dramatically.[66]

Are these particles fecal material from parasites? Are they the debris of degenerated and dying cells? Are they variant (pleomorphic) forms of unfriendly bacteria? We do not know, but Dr. Naessens' work suggests that the presence in blood of many noncellular particles is associated with cancer. They are present to a small degree in the blood of persons who are healthy.

Holistic methods of diagnosis

Should you be seeking treatment with homeopathy or Bach (pronounced "Batch") flower remedies? Your practitioner most likely will spend considerable time asking you questions in order to ascertain your personality, on the basis of which your treatment is selected. Dowsers, relying on the universal knowledge of the unconscious mind, dowse for appropriate remedies. Bach Flower Remedies cannot le

---

[66]Christopher Bird, Gaston Naessens' Symposium on Somatidian Orthobiology: a Beachhead Established, in *The Townsend Letter for Doctors*, October 1991, pp. 797-805.

gally be used as agents for physical healing in the United States.

The effect of homeopathic and Bach flower remedies is to restore emotional/mental balance—and physical balance with it. These remedies so far are without side effects and can be used in conjunction with Western medicine.

Acupuncture is now, usually, included in one's health insurance. This varies by state. In Florida, insurance covers acupuncture treatment if you tell your physician you would like acupuncture and he writes a prescription for it.

Acupuncture is based on the Chinese theory of medicine which in turn is based upon a balance of energies within the body which are referred to as the Five Elements. Traditionally, people get acupuncture at the change of the Five Seasons, recognized in the Orient, so as to stay in balance. Should a person become sick, the acupuncturist pays him or her for not having done his or her work properly.

The acupuncturist diagnoses one's physical condition by taking one's pulse on each wrist, applying three different degrees of pressure while taking the pulse. The quality of pulse at each depth describes the vitality of a particular organ system.

Iridology is an easy way to see your health. With a map of the iris and a mirror, you can assess you own areas of physical strength and weakness.[67] For the sake of objectivity, it is probably better to go to a professional iridologist. However, I do know that black spots on my iris which were present when I had cancer have now faded away.

Early in this century and in the last century, Western physicians as well as Oriental healers were diagnosing people's health by examining their fingernails. It is a neglected art today, but one which can reveal much about not only one's health but one's diet. Are you familiar with white flecks that occur occasionally on a fingernail? Such spots

---

[67]Bernard Jensen, "Iridology Simplified," 1980, Dr. Bernard Jensen, Escondido, California.

can develop as a response to eating large amounts of sugar or other sweets.[68]

To a practiced eye, the skin, hair, body postures, face, tongue and wrinkles all speak of the condition of the internal organs.

Most superficially, dry skin is an indication that the diet is too fatty. The small vessels that nourish and cleanse the skin are blocked and the oil glands are not producing. Excessive consumption of protein is reflected in excessive epidermal growth (protein) which is shed as flaky skin and dandruff. Dandruff is a result of eating too much protein, which makes sense, doesn't it?[69]

Accompanying dry and flaky skin is dry and messy hair. When I had cancer, every day was a "bad hair" day to such an extent that a physician in charge of radiation in her clinical report described me as having "unkempt" hair.

Body postures may be assumed unconsciously in order to relieve pressure on sore or tender organs. For example, a habit of crossing one's legs especially to one side, may indicate that the colic flexure on that side of the body is impacted. I always used to sit with my left leg crossed over my right, possibly indicating an impacted cecum (my appendix, an extension of the cecum, had been removed years before) as has a lumbar subluxation.[70]

Facial wrinkles, if fine and numerous, indicate the excessive consumption of so called (in Oriental medicine) 'expanding' foods such as sweets, coffee and alcohol, while short, deep wrinkles or furrows are the result of excessive consumption of 'contracting' food such as meat, poultry, game fish and fertilized eggs.[71] Either kind of food is extreme and causes one to crave food at the opposite extreme in an effort to find balance. Such cravings are unconscious.

---

[68]Michio Kushi, "How to See Your Health: Book of Oriental Diagnosis," 1980, Japan Publications, Inc., New York and Tokyo.
[69]Kushi, 1980.
[70]Thomas Woleshin, D.C., Fernandina Beach, Florida, Personal communication.
[71]Kushi, 1980.

The condition of the internal organs of the body is mirrored throughout the body: the face, the tongue, the palms, the soles, the ears, etc.

Just as each cell contains in it DNA, which is the master plan for the entire body's growth and development, according to Oriental medicine, each organ has within its form a map of the rest of the body.[72]

The color and texture, swelling or gauntness, edema or firmness of different portions of the face and tongue as well as greasiness, dryness, condition of the pores, all reveal a lot about one's internal organs.

Finally, the voice reveals much about a person's health. A voice can be waterlogged, furry, reedy, thin, bubbly, loud, hearty, penetrating, gravelly, scratchy, etc., all of which carries information to the ears of an experienced diagnostician, and sometimes to those of a layman.

---

[72]See also Okun, M. and Edelstein, L., 1995. The Cell and the Organism: the Role of Subdivisional Cell Replication in the Development and Maintenance of a Multicellular Organism. *Cell Biology International* 19 (10): 851-877.

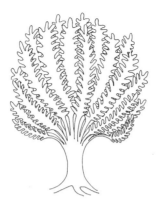

Chapter Six
Do No Harm...

Of the many ways taken by holistic medicine to bring about healing, none of them disobeys the edict contained in the Hippocratic Oath: "Do no harm."

Whatever methods I used for healing did no damage to any cell or to the organization and energy flow of my body, with two exceptions: a diagnostic removal of my breast lumps, and later, a sampling of axillary lymph nodes. I was fortunate to find surgeons who were willing to carry out these surgeries under local anesthetic. These operations traversed my stomach meridian which crosses the breast, and possibly the heart meridian which runs through the armpit. I hope and believe the energy flow through those meridians is healed. Whatever measures I used to heal my troubled physical self only cleaned, nourished and improved it.

The holistic treatments I used were also easy on my pocketbook. Insurance would not have paid for many or all of them then or now. Insurance payments over even a few years would have cost much more than what I spent to heal myself.

The amount I spent on surgery and operating room fees, a weekend "Diet and Cancer" seminar, a new set of pots and pans, four acupuncture treatments, four or five colonic irrigations, and a consultation for some Chinese herbs, were my main expenses over the course of two years. In addition, because I was eating all unprocessed foods, my grocery bill dropped!

What I liked most about my cancer cure is that, just as the Sun shines equally on everyone who is in its path, my preventive and healing lifestyle is equally available and affordable to everyone.

When I had cancer I tried many holistic treatments, but did not take advantage of homeopathy or the Bach Flower Remedies because at the time, I did not know about them. When something was giving good results, such as my diet, I mostly stuck with it and did not replace it with something else. When I was feeling the results of occasionally departing from my healthy way of eating, I used several of the other alternative modalities described briefly below. It is so important to believe in what one is doing and to understand the reasons for it.[73]

I shall begin with the most far out method I tried: radionics. I believe radionics will be the medicine of the future. Light, sound, and aroma therapy, and even herbal and dietary medicine are all part of radionics.

Radionics

Radionics appears to be based on nothing at all. Yet, the practitioner, a traveling man from New Zealand, knew that my vital energy was present in a photograph I sent him. That is why many Native Americans, and many other people, do not like to have their picture taken. Vital energy cannot be accessed or treated through a photocopy of a photograph, as in a newspaper photo.

Upon my photograph the radiologist set the sub-

---

[73]for a recent summary of alternative methods available for treating breast cancer, see Goldberg.

stance bearing the essential energy with which he wanted to treat me. Nearly one hundred miles away, I could feel the energy being broadcast to me. My body felt much stronger over a period of two to three days, and I remained stronger after the treatment. There are those who will say that my improvement was due to the placebo effect (it works because you think it will). However, practitioners of radionics will tell you, its effects are consistent and can be replicated experimentally.

Acupuncture and Chinese herbs

After my breast lump biopsy, a friend with whom I had not spoken in some time chanced to call and speak about the wonderful results she was having from acupuncture. Her call came in an hour before the phone was being disconnected because I was moving to the city. I consulted her acupuncturist very soon after.

This practitioner, although seemingly a caring person, responded not at all to the fact that I had breast cancer. He countered my fear for my life by calmly saying that many people healed themselves through eating macrobiotic or natural vegetarian food, avoiding animal products and processed foods and drinks. One or two hours after lying quietly with painless needles sticking out of me from various places, I noticed that I was feeling well—very well. I felt restored to the level of energy I had before I developed cancer.

I ate more carefully, although I was already eating pretty much the way the acupuncturist had recommended. Although my every level decreased, it did not sink to the lows I had experienced previously.

I had acupuncture only occasionally, sometimes at the change of seasons. Thereby my body maintained itself without my coming to rely on this outside intervention. Acupuncture is, however, along with chiropractic, —and two courses of antibiotics taken when I had not been eating well —the only health treatment I have had for eighteen years.

Several months after my first acupuncture treatment, after carefully following a macrobiotic medicinal diet, I fell off it suddenly by eating a lot of sweets in response to stress which I had not learned to manage. The result was a rapid downward spiral in my energy and mood. Was I back where I had started? Because my descent was so rapid, Michio Kushi referred me to a Chinese herbalist.

The herbs and the profound, intangible help of this practitioner also, restored me to the point that I did not finish taking the second course of herbs. I cannot say more about this treatment except that herbalism is a deep science just as particle physics is. It is true: Nature has given us everything we need to heal ourselves. That is also why the destruction of the natural environments and the irrecoverable loss of thousands of species is a terrible, but ongoing, mistake.

Exercise

Whatever exercise one carries out is important for the circulation of one's body fluids. The return of our venous blood and of our lymphatic fluids from the tissues is carried out passively by the squeezing action of our muscles on our veins and lymphatic vessels. If we exercise, our heart does not have to do all the work in changing venous blood for oxygenated blood at the body's periphery such as in our fingertips and lower limbs.

Especially important news for persons who have cancer is the "strict connection" between regular exercise (a moderate training program two to three times a week for seven months) and the activity of protective natural killer cells observed in 24 women with breast cancer. Their comfort and "satisfaction of life" increased after only five weeks.[74]

---

[74]Peters C., Lotzerich H., Niemeier K., Schule K, Uhlenbruck G.: Influence of a moderate exercise training on natural killer cytotoxicity and personality traits in cancer patients. *Anticancer Res.* May, 1994, 14 (3A): 1033-1036.

Following my diagnosis, after lying around for a month mainly doing nothing because I had become so weak, I realized that I had to resume my habit of walking. Because the temperature in w!estern Massachusetts had been enjoying a cold snap of single numbers in the daytime for nearly a month, I bought snowmobile boots with felt packs inside to keep my feet warm, and again started walking in the snowy woods.

Because I had scarcely any energy in general, I carried out an exercise for gaining energy I had read in one of Lobsang Rampa's books.[75] It was this, best done in sunlight and outside:

First I cleaned out stale air from the bottom and top of my lungs:

Standing with my feet a shoulder width apart, I held my arms in front of me and inhaled all I could. Then I gasped in a tiny bit more. I held my breath as long as I could, then exhaled *against resistance* in four or five short putts until my lungs were empty. Then I breathed normally.

To increase my small store of energy, I followed Rampa's further advice:

I carried out the first part of the breath cleansing exercise. When my lungs were as full as I could make them, I drew my arms back to my shoulders as fast as I could, then pushed them outwards again against as much resistance as I could create, then drew them back again as fast as I could, and so forth until I had done this perhaps six times. (When I started out I could do it only once or twice). Then I exhaled as fast and as deeply as I could and followed this with a second breath cleansing exercise.[76]

Carrying out the above exercises actually got me up and moving about again, although at first I thought I would collapse.

---

[75]Teusday Lobsang Rampa, "Doctor From Lhasa," Corgi, 1980, pp. 201-205.
[76]Rampa, pp. 201-205.

In a temporary network of persons with cancer, I was referred to a man with lung cancer who recommended a trampoline as being unsurpassed for lymphatic return. So I bought one from the local seller of trampolines, the gentleman who with his wife ran the pizza house in an adjoining town. He took me behind the counter to the back of the small building. Behind the swinging doors that led to the kitchen was a small trampoline upon which he cheerfully bounced up and down for a few minutes. It was wonderful, he said, because he was on his feet all day. When he began to feel weary, he jumped on the trampoline a few times and felt completely refreshed.

I loved my trampoline. Four feet across, I kept it in my then-large kitchen and bounced while food was cooking. Sometimes I played music and danced on it.

I have been told and do believe that walking is the best exercise, if you do enough of it. I walked an hour a day, every day, in the country, but when I returned to live in the city, I resumed running. At first I could run only a few hundred feet, then a quarter of a mile. Eventually, I was running two miles a day.

I would recommend Yoga or T'ai Chi to any person with cancer and in general. Through Yoga, one stimulates different organ systems. Doing T'ai Chi naturally stimulates all of one's energy meridians, bringing about balance between the different organ systems.

Hot towel scrub

I was instructed to do this when I had my first macrobiotic dietary consultation. It is part of the routine instruction to persons seeking the beneficial change in lifestyle which Macrobiotics has to offer. I strongly recommend to anyone the summary of dietary, cooking and lifestyle suggestions contained in Michio Kushi's small (64-page) updated booklet, "*Standard Macrobiotic Diet,*"[77] or in

---

[77]1996, One Peaceful World Press, Becket Massachusetts.

his more extensive, "*The Macrobiotic Approach to Cancer.*"[78] It is worth much more than its weight in gold whether you are sick or aiming to stay healthy.

If you wish to study healing with food and lifestyle in greater depth, I enthusiastically refer you to Aveline and Michio Kushi's deeper work, "*Macrobiotic Diet,*"[79] along with many other works on health and the Cosmic Order which are available from the Kushi Institute.

After dipping a washcloth in water as hot as you can stand, scrub every part of your body until the skin is red, starting from the toes and moving upward to heart level, then from the face down to heart level. I was told to do this twice a day. It was an extraordinary experience. Yes, it was time-consuming and yes, it was an uncomfortable prospect when living in New England in midwinter. But my body has rarely felt so comfortable, before or since.

As I scrubbed away, unconsciously I was stimulating acupuncture points which needed it. Afterward, I gratefully found myself in a body which was relaxed so deeply that my mind was calmed also. I felt fortified and strengthened. The troubles of the day and the idea that I had cancer were chased far away by my feelings of well-being.

It is possible that, with the outer layers of skin that were removed twice daily, twenty *per cent.* of the toxins in my body were being removed, leaving my liver and kidneys with much less work to do.

Colonic irrigation

Periodic cleansing of the colon has been practiced since ancient Egyptian times. For meat eaters it is most likely a good idea.

The point of colonic irrigation is to clean out any undigested material which is sticking to the colon's walls and which may have become impacted within the *diverticula*. The *diverticula* are the series of little digestive pouches of which,

[77]Kushi 1991, pp. 40-44.

with its autonomic muscle, the colon is mostly composed.

Occasionally I had colonic irrigation which, had I always been true to my diet, I would not have needed. Colonic irrigation boosts a person's energy because, like the rest of our body, the lining of the colon is connected to all other points within our body. A colonic irrigation is like having acupuncture in the balancing effect it can have on one's organs.

Coffee enemas

Jacqui Davis cured her melanoma with the Gerson Diet and coffee enemas.[79] They are a part of several different alternative therapies for cancer.

Coffee enemas are valuable in removing toxins. When toxins are suddenly released into the bloodstream as the result of a dietary detoxification program or by fasting (not recommended if you have cancer) a person's system is overwhelmed and one can collapse.

Coffee enemas have the advantage of being do-able at home. They flush out the gall bladder and stimulate the liver.

Bonnie Randolph cured her ovarian cancer after surgery, radiation and chemotherapy had failed. She followed the Metabolic Treatment Program of Dr. Nicholas Gonzales in New York. The program included a program of individualized diet and supplements with daily coffee enemas.[80]

Anti parasite program

I did not use Dr. Clark's program to heal myself but I include here a brief summary of her work because I feel it is so important to be aware of the conditions she discusses in her work and of the dangers and commonness of parasites. Unfortunately, we are no longer as aware or educated about

---

[79]Jaquie Davis, 1977, "Cancer Winner," Pacific Press, Pierce City, Missouri.
[79]1991, Return to Life: How I Defied My Doctor and Survived Ovarian Cancer, EastWest Journal, November/December: 52-57.

hygiene as we were in the days before antibiotics.

Hulda Regehr Clark, N.D., used a kind of electric kinesiology in her research. She found that certain kinds of chemicals, especially alcohols and benzenes, may accumulate in organ tissues and allow parasites to become established and multiply there, causing cancer, AIDS, Alzheimer's syndrome, and a host of other chronic diseases, depending on which organs are affected. She prescribes a specific program of herbal combinations to rid the body of parasites and recommends taking two amino acids with the herbal preparations. She also points out what chemicals to avoid in cosmetics, the household environment, and in food and drink.

Her books are detailed with case histories and a remarkable list of common household items which, she says, through their chemical content, particularly of benzenes and propyl alcohol, promote the establishment of parasites. Chemical solvents such as benzenes, propanol, and other alcohols are not found on labels but are present in trace amounts in store-bought bottled water, store-bought fruit juice, cold breakfast cereals and carbonated soft drinks! They are present in most pet foods, in cosmetics, in shampoos, and in laundry detergents. Dr. Clark recommends such measures as brushing one's teeth with baking soda and doing laundry with Borax followed by a rinse to which vinegar has been added.[80] To prevent accumulations of chemical solvents in one's vital organs, it is worthwhile to have one of Dr. Clark's books in hand.

Dr. Clark mentions in her book, "The Cure for All Cancers," that the Macrobiotic Diet, which includes a natural lifestyle, is also effective in ridding the body of parasites.[81]

I personally do not know anyone who has followed Dr. Clark's methods to cure cancer. But I naturally follow the lifestyle recommendations found in her book and which

[80]Clark, 1993. See especially pp. 37, 68-69.
[81]Clark, p.20

accompany a macrobiotic or natural lifestyle.

714-X:

A brief mention of the work of Dr. Gaston Naessens, whose work we mentioned earlier, is included here because, although the man was hounded and prevented from practicing in the United States, his research is being continued by others and may even provide the foundation for a revolution in basic biology.

Developed by Dr. Naessens, 714-X is injected daily for a period of months into the lymph glands of the groin. I suppose that doing such a thing would program into anyone's unconscious mind that they were fighting for his/her life. I could not bear to watch a friend do it. It is not a path I would have taken, as my preference was and is always to stay close to Mother Nature, as close as possible. I have heard of people being cured by following this method but for me, this is hearsay.

A stunning finding by Dr. Naessens is the presence of microscopic particles, "somatids," in the blood, which accompany disease.[82] Whether somatids are cellular waste, viruses or other is unknown at this time as far as I know. Yet, the presence and relative absence of such particles when viewed with a dark field microscope, seem at the very least to be an accurate way to evaluate the progression or remission of cancer. It might be a useful diagnostic tool if used more widely.

Teas

Evidently associated with a lack of alcoholism and cancer in two disparate Russian villages, government researchers tried to find out what these two towns had in common. It proved to be, so the story has it, "tea-kvass," or sugared tea which had been fermented with kombucha

---

[82]Bird, 1991.

mushrooms.[83]

I recently have tried the tea myself and noted that it indeed allows the liver to bounce back quickly from a banquet of eating and drinking. I have heard that long term use of it may damage the kidneys, but this is hearsay. It is not recommended for certain, more *yin* kinds of cancer, such as breast cancer and other peripheral cancers.

Essiac has been termed a "wonder herb" which has helped friends and which evidently continues to help many. Its drawback is that the tea made from this herb must be prepared fresh because it does not keep.[84] However, I have heard that commercial extracts of it are being sold in health stores.

Tea made from a combination of red clover and chaparral was used by Native Americans to purify their system. I drank a good deal of it, especially initially while I was still shopping around for a treatment for my cancer in which I had faith. It seemed to help, but not as much as changing my way of eating eventually did.

Diet

Native Americans and Hawaiians, to protect themselves against the ravages of diabetes, alcoholism, cancer and kidney problems that accompany the Western diet, are returning to their traditional ways of eating and are recovering their health.

For physical recovery from cancer, I feel, because I did well with it and know of many others who have also,[85] that using a macrobiotic, piscovegetarian (fish—not initially! —in small amounts, plus grains, vegetables and a little fruit)

[83]Tom Valentine, Kombucha, a Fermented Beverage With Real 'Zing' In It!, *Search For Health* ! (6), July/Aug. 1993 pp. 1-14.

[84]Richard Thomas, "The Essiac Report," 1993. The Alternative Treatment Information Network (Los Angeles).

[85]See case histories in Kushi, 1991 and in: East West Foundation with Ann Fawcett and Cynthia Smith, "Cancer Free: Thirty Who Healed Themselves Naturally," 21991, Japan Publications, Inc.

diet is crucial. I was managing to hold onto some of my very much diminished vitality by giving up coffee and meat, fowl and dairy products. But I did not notice a definite improvement in my physical condition and level of energy until I went on my particular diet of whole foods.

People have used several different diets to cure themselves of cancer.

There is the grape diet which, the author says, is for people on whom doctors have given up hope.[86] A former teacher of mine, the late Frances Sakoian, told me that she had seen a remarkable cancer cure by going on the Grape Diet with a friend who was sick. That is all I know about it. The book about the Grape Diet was written by Doctor Johanna Brandt, a South African naturopath who, having healed herself with this diet, came to the United States to share her information with other people. Her little book is convincing reading and therefore recommended.

The Gerson Diet originated in Germany. The best layman's testimonial to it that I know is Jacqui Davis's book "Cancer Winner," about her recovery from advanced malignant melanoma, without radiation or chemotherapy, by means of the Gerson Diet.

One difficulty about following the Gerson Diet is that it requires fresh calves' liver juice. Juicing liver is something that requires a hydraulic press (as in a Norwalk Juicer), which is very costly indeed. But the Gerson diet, with coffee enemas and the loving support of her husband, not only saved her life but restored Jacquie Davis to radiant health. Her hair, which had become grey, turned dark again, her nails grew long and her skin became smooth and radiant.[87]

The Raw Foods Diet as a cure for cancer was pioneered by Dr. Ann Wigmore, who founded the Hippocrates

---

[86]Dr. Johanna Brandt, 1989: "How to Conquer Cancer, Naturally," Tree of Life Publications, Palm Springs California. First published 1929 with original title: "The Grape Cure."
[87]Davis, *op. cit.*

Institute for Health in Boston. Dr. Wigmore had noticed that animals of all kinds eat fresh grass when they are not feeling well. When she became sick she healed herself with raw foods and grasses. This she evolved into a program of raw food supplemented with the juice of fresh-grown wheat grass and the fermented water in which whole wheat berries had been soaked.[88]

I have grown and used wheat grass and fermented soak-water myself and found them potent and beneficial. But I have found that the best thing I can do for my body— and every body is different (but how different is not known), is to stick to the way of eating which cured my cancer. As mentioned, that way of eating is the Macrobiotic diet, an Oriental variant of eating the way the Native Americans ate. Because of my personal experience and that of others known to me, I shall discuss it in greater detail below.

Before leaving the subject of diet and cancer I must first mention the forty-two-day fast, supplemented with herbs and juices, used by the late Austrian naturopath, Rudolph Breuss. His book is remarkable reading and contains not only much useful information one can apply oneself but what I consider a valuable list of resources.[89]

Meditation

Visualization is a form of meditation which is of great value to enhance immune system function. This work was pioneered by the Simontons who found that by doing different visualizations, people increased their white cell count and reduced their cancers.[90]

Meditation can be of great importance in safeguarding one against denial, which is a reaction to fear and anxiety. It can be most helpful in relieving anxiety. It can promote a positive outlook. It can also be used to program oneself to do whatever one wants. I carried out different

[88]Ann Wigmore, "The Wheatgrass Diet", 1985, Avery .
[89]Breuss, Rudolph, "The Breuss Cancer Cure", 1995 *alive* books, Burnaby, B.C.
[90]Simonton et al.

meditations for all of the above purposes, as well as other practices with meditation for the sake of my emotional, mental and spiritual outlook.[91] I consider them so important that I shall say more about some of them later in this book and in the future.

Dreams

What can I say, but try to understand them. It is true that there are "false dreams", caused mostly by eating the wrong food at the wrong time, but the dreams of the very sick are especially important. When I had cancer I dreamed frequently and, perhaps because I was looking for it, nearly every dream told me something helpful about my life and which direction to go in. Other persons with cancer, both known to me and about whom I have read, have had dreams that were major guidance for them.[92]

Attitude

Someone once said that life is a series of attitudes. Does this mean that if you have no attitudes you have no life? It might mean this because without any attitudes you might be too good for this world. But some attitudes raise us up and improve our existence.

It is important to realize that as one pursues a more natural way of eating and lifestyle, many negative feelings will gradually melt away. Unfortunately, our feelings when we are sick may prevent this or make persistence difficult. Such feelings, which would be termed "maladaptive" by physicians and nurses, can be dealt with in a roundabout way. For more on this subject, see Chapter Ten.

---

[91]Milo, 1996a.
[92]Antonia G. Milo. Bridging Worlds: Decision Making of Individuals with Cancer or AIDS, *Proc. 1nt. Conf. Shamanism and Alt. Modes of Healing.*1995, pp. 272-274.

Compatibilities of the above with Western Medicine

The above methods which I used to heal myself, namely: radionics, acupuncture, exercise, hot towel scrub, meditation with other spiritual practices and the macrobiotic diet are, as far as I know, without negative side effects and are compatible with surgery, radiation and chemotherapy. I had surgery: a diagnostic excision biopsy, before changing the way I ate. I did not have radiation or chemotherapy, so I can only report what others have told me firsthand about their experience.

Speaking generally, people I know who were on the Macrobiotic Diet seemed to recover more quickly than expected from surgery. I do not know about radiation, but with chemotherapy there occurred some nausea but not the anticipated vomiting and diarrhea.

To my knowledge, none of the holistic methods of healing cited above, with the exception of *kombucha* mushroom tea, damages the body in any way on a short or long-term basis.

Having some familiarity with medical terminology and ways, I inquired of my physicians about the long-term effects of chemotherapy and radiation.

I found out that chemotherapy would temporarily erase my immune system (the body's first defence against foreign matter such as cancer cells). I was told that radiation of my breast would leave it drawn up like a fried egg against my chest and also would damage my lungs so that I might not breathe as well in the future.

Because I had been forcing myself to run again, and I did not want a treatment that would damage my body, radiation ceased to be an option. I was told that with radiation in later years, around the age of eighty, I might—"if you live that long"—develop lung cancer, "but by then it won't matter." What! Did I want to get cancer all over again? Certainly

61

it would "matter"!

Anyone should feel free to ask his/her physician or holistic practitioner for the explanations he or she needs, and to change physician/pracititioner if not satisfied with the answers given. Many physicians are more forthcoming with information now than they were.

According to a well-known holistic physician, radiation and chemotherapy are not only crude ways to treat people but will be obsolete before long.[93] Perhaps they are obsolete now! Unfortunately, systematic records of holistic healings are few.

The persons I know who survived cancer with radiation and chemotherapy seem to show us that in curing and in healing, the bottom line is: what is our Soul's intent?[94] For it will be served.

[93]Andrew Weil, M.D.,"Spontaneous Healing", 1995, Fawcett Columbine, 1995, p.268.
[94]Stylianos Atteshlis, Ph.D., D.D., M.Psy., M.Mcs., General Lecture Series, Strovolos, Cyprus.

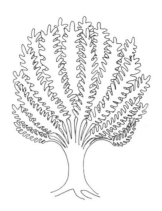

Chapter Seven
Helping Life to Heal

One reason why it was so helpful when my father kept telling me: "Take your time", when I had cancer, was because to take *my* time meant that I had a choice.

Having power in a situation is about having choice. Our choices are not simply about which direction to go in or what treatment to choose. They are also about how fast or slow we want to go. To choose my treatment at my own rate of thinking (slow) removed the pressure of having to make up my mind without having enough information. So I waited... continuing to seek, pray and meditate... and weeks turned into months.

Eventually I realized that endless waiting, not trusting the results of my mammogram, could also prove to be Denial, the ostrich's method of coping with danger. So I decided to have the lump in my breast removed for diagnosis. A look at the tumor cells under a microscope would tell the story. If the diagnosis was malignant, then I would have to get moving and do something. I would no longer be able to say to myself that my mammogram and thermogram were perhaps not one hundred *per cent.* accurate and that maybe I did not have "cancer." I thought I would know for certain after surgery if I had "cancer" or not, even though I had been experimenting with vegetarian eating, doing my daily meditations and exercising.

I wanted the surgery done under a local anesthetic because I felt I would have less pain afterwards and also, so that I could be sure, because of my own dread of mutilation, to keep my breast.

The loss of one's entire breast, even if to save one's life, may cause profound grief and, later, rage that may be repressed. Neither emotion helps the immune system, nor does mastectomy benefit the body's natural flow of energy through the acupuncture meridians. However, some women have been cured and survived it well, knowing that a mastectomy cannot remove their essence nor mutilate their "dream body" or their soul.

Excision biopsy (lumpectomy) with radiation has for some time been recognized as a treatment for breast cancer which is as beneficial as mastectomy. Perhaps the day will come when surgery—and radiation—will be avoided altogether! A beginning has been made.

The surgeon I found who would operate under a local anesthetic was a country surgeon who was much loved by all his patients. He prayed unobtrusively before he began to cut. From his demeanor during the surgery I knew that my diagnosis was malignant. After it was over, he allowed me to examine the two lumps with tentacles to which healthy tissue was attached.

The whole thing was painless, and relatively cheap. I had no medical insurance and in 1981, the surgeon's fee with the operating room fee was six hundred dollars—very little compared to what years of insurance premiums would have cost me... I felt very fortunate to have savings.

After leaving the hospital, I filled a prescription for painkillers I never needed, drove myself to lunch in a restaurant I liked some forty miles away and returned home to nap. An ordinary, sterile rubber band was left hanging out at the end of my incision so the wound could drain. After two days, the rubber band and later, the clamps that held the wound

64

together were removed.

I consulted a Professor Emeritus at Harvard Medical School who was an authority on breast cancer. He had written a book about it and insisted that his patients read the book. The good part was, the book explained all the treatments and acquainted you with what to expect. The bad part was that of the few cases, described in depth, all died within a few years.[95] That was 1981. The outlook for breast cancer is *much* better now.

Before and after my surgery I had been reading about people who cured themselves of cancer with diet. Then I moved to the city because I expected to take both radiation and chemotherapy and I wanted the most up to date treatment with the best equipment. In the city, not long after my surgery, a friend told me about a Diet and Cancer seminar being given one weekend by the Kushi Institute. I attended it

After learning about theory from Ed Esko and Dr. Marc Van Caughenberg, and about macrobiotic cooking methods from Aveline Kushi, I had a dietary consultation with Michio Kushi. Convinced by everything they had said, I immediately began to eat a natural diet that was limited to certain foods because of my serious condition. It took me about two weeks to learn how to prepare medicinal meals which I found absolutely delicious.

If you entrust part or all of your healing to a way of life, the first thing you want to know is if it worked for anyone else. I asked for and was given the telephone number of a woman who had had breast cancer, which spread to her colon. That was two years previous and she was fine. I heard about and met some other people who had been cured of different kinds of cancer through natural eating and lifestyle.[96]

Then I consulted doctors at two leading medical

---

[95]Oliver Cope, M.D., "The Breast", 1974, Little Brown.
[96]East West Foundation with Ann Fawcett and Cynthia Smith.

centers in New England. They recommended to me a combination of chemotherapy and radiation. I also consulted a holistic medical doctor who also recommended conventional medical treatment. But he spoke to me as an equal and a friend. There was a picture over his desk of a bird flying and a quote from "Jonathan Livingston Seagull". It was a message for me. The quote was: "They fly because they think they can."

This doctor asked me to make self portraits and other drawings which were revealing. His interpretations of them gave me insight about my need to give to others and to society.

By taking my time, I decided not to have radiation, or chemotherapy, nor the mastectomy that had originally been recommended by two surgeons.

I realized, as I continued following my natural way of eating, that for three years before I was diagnosed with cancer, a voice in my head used to say to me, at intervals, "Eat the way the Indians ate."

While having buttered toast with jelly with my morning coffee, I would think about how the Native Americans ate. They ate no butter and very little fat because game and wild fowl are not very fatty, occasional meat, no coffee, no jams and jellies. No, I did not want to eat the way the Native Americans ate, at all.

Edgar Cayce reiterated that it's not what enters our mouth but what leaves our mouth that pollutes us.[97] This is certainly true because what we are is so much more than our physical body. It is so easy when living in a materialistic time and place to identify ourselves with our fleshly garment.

Yes, we human beings can and do eat everything from the animal and vegetable kingdoms. But, let us look at this body of ours a little more closely.

---

[97]Read et. Al.

Diet and the Human Form

Not only has archaeology uncovered evidence that early man ate mainly vegetables, but traditional peoples of the earth today, aside from those who inhabit the extreme climates of the circumpolar regions, also are mainly vegetarian with whole grains being the staff of life.

Different kinds of animals and human beings differ markedly not only in the form and number of their teeth but in the length of the intestines as well. A comparison of human teeth with the teeth of different animals: meat eaters, vegetable eaters, and fruit eaters shows a resemblance closest to the animals that live principally on vegetables and fruits. A classic herbivore such as a rabbit has about twenty two feet of intestine. A cat, by contrast, has about seven feet of intestine. We humans have intestines that are about thirteen feet long. Length of the intestine is related to the time necessary for optimal digestion of the kinds of food for which one's body is best adapted.[98] Based on the number and form of our teeth and on the length of our intestines, humanity falls somewhere between animals that live on fruit and those that live on vegetables including grains.[99]

Animal foods have become a dietary staple for (some) humans only recently: a few thousand years ago. "That's not nearly enough time to evolve new mechanisms to give us protection from those kinds of foods."[100]

Why has the food-to-feces transit time more than tripled since the turn of the last century?[101] Can you imagine having the same food stay in your intestines for nearly three days?

A vegetarian diet, which includes grains, vegetables, beans and fruits is evidently the most natural diet for man as stated above (see Chapter Four).

---

[98]Kushi, 1991, p.25.

[99]Swami Sri Yukteswarji, "The Holy Science", Self Realization Fellowship, 1990 (eighth edition), pp. 62-67.

[100]Campbell.

[101]Goldberg, p. 78

How diet can heal

If someone puts sugar in your car's gas tank, the car is not going to recover. But if we stop putting excessive amounts of food in our bodies that it was not designed to digest, we improve. If we are seriously sick and change our diet to eat very simply and very low on the food chain, it is logical for us to improve. Hippocrates, the father of modern medicine, said to "Treat food as medicine and medicine as food." [101]

Sickness is a manifestation of one or more diseased organ systems which can have stress lifted from them by a medicinal diet.

Our organ systems work together as a whole, each organ maintaining its functions within a certain range of values. Because of this characteristic of self maintenance, called *homeostasis,* our body temperature maintains itself within a wide range of temperature in the outside environment. Because of homeostasis the level of acidity in our blood varies little, no matter how much alcohol or orange juice we may drink. The saltiness of our blood remains about the same, whatever we eat. Our kidneys will maintain our blood and body fluids at a fairly constant volume and concentration while the liver and gall bladder regulate the toxin, sugar and fat content of our blood. The pancreas along with the liver maintains our blood sugar level.

As they do their work, our different organs function not chaotically but rhythmically. The prime example is our heart.

Our diaphragm has an innate rhythm which we can override through an act of will if we choose to do so. Our intestines move the food along with gentle, rhythmic contractions. The cells of our organs carry out metabolic, and especially obvious in the case of sex cells, replicating activ-

---

[101] Yet it is relatively recent that nutritional teaching has become part of a medical student's curriculum.

ity according to a rhythm. Our body rhythms are regulated unconsciously in a God and Nature given way.

The rhythms of our organ functions are also homoeostatically controlled. That is, these rhythms may vary, but not too much. Let us consider our heart. The heart beat in an adult is usually between sixty and eighty beats a minute. If a person sleeps poorly and takes several tranquil-lizers to go to sleep, his or her heart rate may drop below this range as he or she falls into a drugged sleep. If a per-son who is out of shape lifts a heavy object or tries to move a piano, his or her heartbeat may soon become very rapid.

The range between the slowest and fastest rhythm, for example, at which an organ functions normally, is its 'wave envelope'. Our organs do not perform as efficiently with rhythms or quantities of biochemical reactions which take place outside their own "wave envelope" of innate parameters.

When we eat simple food or a healing diet, one to which our body is well adapted, our organs do not have to go to extremes to do their work. Instead of extremes of function and recovery, our organs function within a narrow wave envelope that places minimal stress on them .

The function of our organs is interconnected. To help part of the body is to help the whole of it. By relieving the stress on the digestive organs, liver and kidneys, the rest of the body, and with it, the personality, is relieved of much stress also. That is in part how a natural, healing way of eating works.

A healing diet also works by helping the body to eliminate toxins and fats as well as by providing plenty of nourishing food.

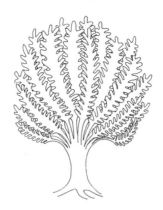

Chapter Eight
The Way the Native Americans Ate

After I was well launched into the Macrobiotic Diet, I found that I was eating just about the way the Native Americans ate, after all.

The Macrobiotic Diet is a set of principles of eating and cooking which, applied in a certain time and place, resulted in the foods and cooking methods now known popularly as "macrobiotic". As a way of eating in the modern world it was brought to the West from Japan by the late George Ohsawa, and his students, Aveline and Michio Kushi and Cornelia and the late Herman Aihara. Ohsawa, had cured himself of tuberculosis by eating the way vegetarian Zen Buddhist monks had traditionally eaten.[103]

What the Macrobiotic Diet refers to is not the vegetarian style of cooking of one particular culture, but eating close to nature in whatever natural environment you may be: that is, eating regionally and seasonally, eating fresh, unprocessed foods without additives, eating low on the food chain, with occasional meat or fish as occurred in a traditional society that lived modestly and close to the earth. It means cooking in stainless steel, iron or earthen pots and

---

[103]George Ohsawa, "Macrobiotics - the Way of Healing". 1981. George Ohsawa Foundation Press, Oroville CA.

pans, and over flame rather than with electricity.

I strongly recommend reading at least the booklet written by Michio Kushi[104] to anyone who is interested in better health and a happier lifestyle. (It is filled with information in simple list form, including basic recipes). What is presented here is bare bones. For those who wish to read deeper and to understand the basis of oriental medicine, the cosmology that underlies macrobiotics as medicinal food as well as more about macrobiotic cooking, I strongly recommend reading "Macrobiotic Diet," by Michio and Aveline Kushi.[105] It is a golden book with a silver cover.

Eating close to nature, our diet varies from season to season, according to climate, and when used medicinally is corrected for when you were born, your age, your gender, and other personal factors. It is a way of eating that is relatively low in protein. Protein comes mostly from grain, beans and vegetables and is sufficient.

Our teeth are fine grinders of grain. When I consulted Michio Kushi I was told, roughly, that more than half my food should be whole grains. When well, I also eat pita bread, - not much - corn tortillas, and pasta. I eat a higher proportion of whole grain in winter than in summer. I was told when sick to eat one bowl of brown rice a day as part of my intake of whole grains. Had I been Native American, I would have been eating corn, wild rice or amaranth instead of rice with my other mainstays being beans and squash.

I eat small amounts of beans cooked with seaweeds. Small amounts of seaweeds not only provide many minerals that may have been missing from our diet, but provide iodine which is necessary for thyroid function.[106] For while I was sick, I was told to eat beans that were not fatty: lentils, chickpeas and aduki beans. You would be surprised how

---

[105]Edited by Alex Jack. Japan Publications, Inc., Tokyo and New York, 1985.
[106]Hypothyroidism and a slow metabolism are associated with breast cancer. Dr. Neal Barnard points out that eating complex carbohydrates increases your metabolism (pp. 94-96).

much beans can vary in their fat content! I also learned that cooking beans gently with seaweed will make them delicious and of a texture not obtainable in any other way that I know of. Furthermore, it seems to eliminate gas.

About one quarter to one third of my intake was to be vegetables with emphasis on the family of vegetables called "cruciferae" (cabbage, Brussels sprouts, broccoli, cauliflower, collards). I was told to avoid vegetables of the nightshade family (potatoes, tomatoes, peppers, zucchini, eggplant). As a result, I now rarely want to eat any of the nightshades. One's tastes change. It was winter squash, not zucchini, that was a staple of the Native American, as it is of the Japanese Macrobiotic, diet.

Proteinases are enzymes we secrete that break down the proteins we eat. Grains and legumes/beans are high in *proteinase inhibitors*, which means that they do not mix well with eating meat, fowl or other high protein foods. The Macrobiotic Diet is helpful to people with AIDs, which is interesting as they are now treating AIDs patients with synthetic proteinase inhibitors.

The rest of what I ate, aside from snacks, condiments and pickles, were one or two small bowls of lightly flavored miso soup a day.

At this point, as a westerner, I must sing the praise of miso. Miso is fermented soybean paste with sea salt. You make soup by adding about one quarter of a teaspoon per cup to the water in which you have boiled or steamed some vegetables. I add it to the water by creaming it against the side of the pot, then stirring it into the liquid but it is more properly made by dissolving the miso in a small amount of hot liquid and then adding this to the rest.

Miso soup tastes somewhat like the best quality of beef bouillon and gives to vegetable broth or soup a rich, meaty quality that even beef bouillon can't produce. It is the way I always wanted beef bouillon to taste.

There are many kinds of miso but I used *mugi* miso

(barley miso), which is a good, middle of the road miso for a person who is sick.

On my diet I could, as I got healthier, occasionally eat some fish but not the meaty, big game fish. I also avoided shellfish - clams, oysters, mussels, shrimp, lobsters for some time, as these are bottom scavengers and hard on the liver. To supplement whole beans/legumes as a source of protein, I sometimes eat tofu and other soy products. When sick with cancer, I was told to avoid tofu as it is processed and instead, to eat tempeh.

Tempeh is partly crushed whole soybeans which have been made into a cake and lightly fermented, a kind of soybean cheese. It originated in Indonesia. I now prefer it to tofu and my cats love it also. Seitan or "wheatmeat" made from wheat gluten is another source of protein.

Homemade salt or rice bran pickles, pickled sauerkraut, and macrobiotic specialties such as salted plums (umeboshi), pickled ginger and pickled daikon (large white radish) pickles are all recommended to help the digestive process and to remove animal fat from the system.

You can read about condiments in "Standard Macrobiotic Diet". Instead of putting a pat of butter or oleomargarine on my grains or vegetables, I most often use toasted sesame seeds ground up with sea salt. This seasoning is called *gomashio* or "sesame salt". The ratio of seeds to salt depends on your physical condition. Sometimes I use lemon juice or delicious Japanese salted plum (umeboshi) vinegar. Fine quality soy sauce, without preservatives, has a bouquet like fine wine. I used it to season food while cooking, not sloshed on afterward. All salt that is used is sea salt, the salt which has the same mineral composition as our blood.

Beverages are mainly teas or drinks for specific physical conditions. The most usual drink is the roasted twig tea (kukicha) which is the staple drink in China and Japan. It has scarcely any caffeine and its flavor is pleas antly robust. It can be supplemented with green tea, roasted barley tea, dandelion root tea or grain coffee of which there are several, Roma being the brand most commonly found in supermarkets.

Cooking methods most often involve steaming, boiling, water sauteing or cooking "waterless" in their own juice in a heavy pot with a lid. In cold and temperate climates, pressure cooking is often resorted to although this cannot be "the way the Native Americans ate". For a sick person, pressure cooked grain can be very helpful, healthful and healing. If you are sick it can be very comforting to know the reasons that underlie whatever method of healing you may choose. If you are considering healing yourself with alternative methods, it may relieve your mind and you may find comfort in the more detailed information contained in "Macrobiotic Diet" by Michio and Aveline Kushi[107]. It is the only way of eating I can think of for which the reasons are so coherent and comprehensive.

There are rules to be observed whether eating the way the Native Americans ate or a "macrobiotic" diet. The main rules are to eat fresh food rather than food which has been processed or preserved (I eat no canned or frozen foods except, occasionally, for example, sardines or olives), to eat foods which grow regionally, to eat foods that are in season, and to eat foods whole: stems as well as leaves, peels as well as flesh, to eat the whole fruit or vegetable rather than to drink the juice.[108]

---

[107]1985. Japan Publications.

[108]It may be helpful, especially when eating produce that has not been organically grown, to wash it to remove pesticide residues. You can soak vegetables and fruits for ten minutes in water to which a small amount of Chlorox has been added, and then rinse and soak another ten minutes in water, or use "Clean Greens" vegetable wash which you can request in health food stores if they do not carry it.

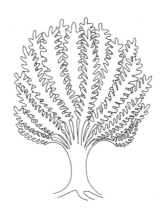

Chapter Nine
Personal Experiences

I found that there were several 'minuses' and 'pluses' in eating close to nature, especially as austerely as the healing diet that was prescribed for me nearly twenty years ago. The biggest minus is the big question that eating in this way asks of us: Do we live to eat or do we eat to live? There you have it. As time passes, the food tastes increasingly delicious!

Minuses
A diet that is close to Nature takes getting used to. But now it is easy and my preferred way of eating. I feel better and have more energy if I follow it pretty closely. Fortunately, one's sense of taste seems to change when one has been eating in this way long enough, so that everything is a pleasure to eat. One's taste becomes more delicate, more subtle.

A medicinal diet can be isolating. I could no longer go, as had been my wont, to a diner for coffee and a donut to read the newspaper during leisure time. Going out to eat was difficult too. Fortunately, with the semi-revolution in America's dietary consciousness, it is now usually possible to eat and to eat well when I go out to dinner. One reason for this may be that I now live in the South where people understand, or used to understand, food and vegetables and where they serve the grits I ate since childhood.

Another minus is that eating closer to nature is time consuming. You don't open a can or pop a TV dinner in the microwave. In fact, you never use a microwave. Instead, you wash and cut vegetables and cook them yourself. Grain and especially, beans, can take some time to cook, time during which one may also do something else. I find it is best, two or three mornings a week, to cook a two or three day's supply of rice and another grain and a bean and a vegetable dish which will last for about three meals.

Initially, and it can be an unpleasant experience, one's body makes the change from a protein to a complex carbohydrate[109] economy. During this transitional time, I felt that I was "running on empty", like a car that had no gas left in the tank but which was still, somehow, continuing to move.

For two years, as my body went through healing changes, I was what some people called 'emaciated'. I was not wasting away from disease. I was detoxifying. Then I gained weight and returned to "normal".

The Greeks say that "There is no good without bad and no bad without good." Just as there were minuses, so also were there and are there pluses to eating in a way that is as close to Nature as possible.

Pluses

The first plus is that, when one's body is running on a complex carbohydrate economy, one can go for a long time and even miss a meal without being hungry.

The second has to do with nuclear radiation. A scientist whose laboratory was near the epicenter of the blast at Hiroshima instructed his co-workers to eat whole brown rice only, with vegetables, beans, seaweed and to take miso

---

[109]Complex carbohydrates, unlike simple ones (sugars) must be broken down (digested) before they can be absorbed into the blood.

soup. These people, who returned to eating traditionally instead of consuming the modern polished white rice, had no radiation sickness![110]

Another plus is that with the change in the way food tastes, one becomes more intuitive about what foods are good for one. One automatically recovers the awareness that little children have of what food is good for them.

One of the two fundamental pluses I noted was mood change. No longer did I have periods of depression, deeply sad feelings that were not necessarily related to my menstrual cycle. My mood became steadier and calmer.

What happened? I was no longer a victim of the "Sugar Blues," well named by author William Dufty.[111] I ceased to have cravings for sweets. Evidently food cravings are a symptom of being allergic to that food.

Refined sugar is damaging in many ways.[112] George Ohasawa relates how he went to Africa to see Albert Schweitzer's hospital in Lambarene.[113] Dr. Schweitzer was away, but when George Ohsawa asked the lepers about their diet, he found that it was no longer a traditional one but included large amounts of refined white sugar. He told the lepers to stop eating sugar and to chew their food at least twenty times with each bite. At the end of a few weeks, before he left, there was substantial improvement in the lepers who had followed his advice.

I certainly had craved and eaten a lot of sugar myself with the results of intermittent depression. I was not the only one.

Once a young woman called me and began to unload her tale of woe. She hated and wanted to leave her job, and she wanted to divorce her husband because they were not

---

[110]Tatsuichiro Akizuki, 1981: "Nagasaki 1945", Quartet Books, London, cited in Noboru B. Muramoto, 1988: "Natural Immunity: Insights on Diet and AIDS", George Ohasawa Macrobiotic Foundation, Oroville CA, p. 6.
[111]"Sugar Blues", 1993, Warner Books (reissue). Originally published 1976.
[112]Muramoto, Chapter Four: Sugar, pp. 61-75. Everyone should read this chapter.
[113]Ohsawa.

compatible, yet she needed to work and she didn't know where to go. She also had had a very difficult childhood, and at this point she broke down and started weeping more and more. When she calmed down slightly, I asked her what she ate during the days and at her meals. It turned out she was eating and snacking on a lot of foods that had a high content of sugar. I suggested she leave off eating any kind of sugar for two weeks and then to call me back. But after a week had passed, I saw this same woman in a line outside a movie theater. She was beautifully dressed and holding her husband's arm. She was smiling.

One craves sugars and/or alcohol less when eating smaller amounts of flesh, poultry or even fish and salt.

Thorough chewing makes one's food taste sweeter.[114] It is amazing how sweet certain vegetables and grains, such as carrots, onions, winter squash and rice are!

Another plus about the diet I follow is that the lecithin in the soy products I use helps to remove accumulations of animal fat from the body, as does daikon, the long, fat white radish that is part of the traditional macrobiotic menu. This way of eating could be good for what ails you.

Another minor but perhaps major plus, when I think of the time it saves (if one does not use a dishwasher), is that dishwashing is easy! It is more like dish rinsing. There is no animal fat to cling to the dishes, to the sink, or to you. A comparison of dishwashing labor involved when eating a modern or a traditional diet suggests that animal fat must cling wherever it may be, inside of us or out!

The greatest plus about the way I eat was this: Every time I chopped a vegetable, prepared a soup or cooked some grain, I was saying by my actions to my unconscious mind: "I want to heal. I want to heal. I want to heal." I was reprogramming myself. I was also giving myself confidence as every action also said: "I'm doing this myself! I'm doing this myself! I'm doing this myself!"

---

[114]Kushi, 1985, p. 200.

Perhaps eating close to nature is how people will eat in the Third Millennium. I hope so. The average family in Costa Rica, which exports beef to the United States, eats less meat than the average American housecat.[115] By eating the way the great majority of the world eats, if they are so fortunate as to have food, we unite ourselves with them in a brotherhood, which in the future of Humanity will surely come.

Eating meals

It is very helpful if a sick family member shares his or her approach to food with other members of the family. It is most valuable for family members to support the one who is sick by sharing new taste experiences - and the sacrifice of fond old habits.[116] There is also a strong benefit as people who eat the same way acquire a similar outlook. It may sound far fetched to most westerners, but according to my observation of others and my own experience this is true.

They say that the family that prays together, stays together, but I would say: "The family that eats and prays together, plays and stays together." If we eat good food that we have prepared ourselves, only when we are hungry, we have a pleasant, warm feeling in our stomach and we are grateful. Vacuuming up our food during spare moments in the course of a busy day is not a good attitude to bring to what is, together with breathing, our most intimate act of communion with the world outside our bodies. Eating involves appreciation for the food, for the fact that we have the food, and for the way our body feels.

I had a habit of gulping and running. How to slow down enough to convert to Eating from eating? The answer is very simple. It is *chewing*.[117]

---

[115]Robbins, p. 35.
[116]Kushi, 1991, pp. 154-55.
[117]Kushi, 1985, p. 234

Chewing

A few months after my initial diagnosis I had my first of five dietary consultation with Michio Kushi. He told me to chew each mouthful of food one hundred times. I found it difficult to believe my ears. He said that if I counted the number of times I chewed, chewing each mouthful one hundred times would soon become automatic. He was right.

I now chew about twenty times a mouthful, sometimes more.

When George Ohsawa went to Lambarene and saw the lepers, in addition to not eating sugar, he also told them to chew their food thirty times each mouthful. Why is that?

The secretions of our digestive system becomes increasingly acid from mouth to rectum. The saliva is alkaline. By combining it thoroughly with our food, *and* drink, we alkalinize the contents of our digestive system which is evidently beneficial, as disease or toxic conditions are associated with acidity and the formation of acid within the body.[118][119][120]

Edgar Cayce said: "If an alkalinity is maintained within the system, - especially with the lettuce, carrots and celery - these in the blood supply will maintain such a condition as to immunize a person," and "Cold cannot - does not exist in alkalies."[121] Edgar Cayce, as does macrobiotics or any way of eating close to nature, stressed eating foods grown regionally. Much can be learned from Edgar Cayce.

By maintaining a more alkaline condition within the body, our resistance to infection and disease increases. I have heard many people eating macrobiotically say that they always used to catch cold in winter but that they never do since they changed their way of eating. I myself ceased completely to feel the chill of New England winters.

---

[118]Aihara.
[119]See also Muramoto, Chapter Nine: Chewing, pp. 141-152.
[120]Read *et al.*
[121]Read *et al.*, p. 25.

People who are confident that they are doing a good job of eating naturally are not afraid of disease. They are not afraid of getting AIDS or other communicable diseases and may work closely with persons with AIDS. Eating macrobiotically has also substantially helped people who have AIDS.[122] On the other hand, one woman cured herself of AIDS without eating macrobiotically. She followed her intuition and ate a cleansing diet.[123]

AIDS

Muramoto points out an historical association that is worldwide between eating meat and the incidence of plagues and AIDS.[124]

I believe that no disease need be "terminal", but, as a result of knowing several people who died with AIDS and by losing a friend whom I shall always miss to AIDS, I have also come to believe that there is a mind set associated with AIDS just as there is a mind set associated with cancer. Changing to a natural (macrobiotic) way of eating and lfestyle can do much to improve one's outlook and the way one feels.

Love your skin

When trying to heal oneself by eating naturally, I was told it is important to wear natural fabrics that allow the skin to breathe.[125] The importance of air on one's skin had been neglected compared to what it used to be. Benjamin Franklin himself used to sit naked by his window taking the air, causing a minor scandal as our ambassador in Paris

[122]Michio Kushi and Martha C. Cotrell, M.D. with Mark N. Mead, 1990: "AIDS, Macrobiotics and Natural Immunity, Japan Publication, Inc., Tokyo and New York. This book includes recipes and interviews.
[123]Niro Markoff Asistent, 1991: Why I survive AIDS. New Age Magazine, October, p. 41. Adapted from 1991: "Why I Survive AIDS", Simon & Schuster/Fireside.
[124]Muramoto.
[125]Kushi, 1991, p.41

where I guess they didn't know a lot about that kind of hygiene at the time.

Common experiences

In beginning to eat close to nature, especially if one is making a drastic change and is following one's new diet carefully, one may feel worse in some ways. This can last for a week to two months. I noticed blurry vision for a few weeks in addition to a terrible feeling that I was "running on empty" like a car with no gas in the tank which was somehow continuing to move. I also had some eruptions come and go on my skin. At one point, when abstaining completely from sugar, including dried fruit, I had night sweats for a month.

I lectured and assisted people with self healing meditations for a while at a macrobiotic study center in Brookline. I noticed that persons with cancer who arrived weak and ashen, after a week of total immersion in cooking and eating,[126] left with roses in their cheeks and standing straight instead of bent over. In other words, after only a week, in most cases - those in which sickness was not too advanced or those who had little or no other cancer therapies - there was not only a noticeable but remarkable difference.

Do it?

If you are considering changing diets and lifestyles, especially if you want to try a macrobiotic lifestyle, you may want to call the Kushi Institute. Someone will faithfully return your call to tell you of macrobiotic resources: stores, cooks, counselors and individuals in your area. Here is a warning: some practitioners prescribe the macrobiotic diet without sufficiently understanding the comprehensive theory on which its use as a medicinal diet is based. I am thinking of one tragic case in particular. A woman had been eating in a

---

[126]Milo, 1996a, pp. 5-6.

way recommended by an alleged macrobiotic counsellor. She and her trusting husband had been told that she could have a little turkey breast, two or three times a week, with tragic consequences. So I recommend, if you are sick, that you enquire closely about a person's credentials: whether or not they have studied at the Kushi Institute or the Vega Center.

When I wanted to heal myself I naturally wanted to speak to someone else who had done so. I was soon given the name of a woman whose breast cancer had spread to her colon two years before. She said she was healthy and was very matter of fact about the whole thing. Shared experiences are very comforting and supportive, for if someone else can do it, so can you, if it is your soul's desire.

"Cancer" support groups

I did not attend any. I was so determined to heal myself, God willing, that I did not want to participate in any group that supported the fact that I had "cancer". I refused to think of myself as a "cancer" patient, and even more so, as a "cancer" victim. Yes, I felt like a victim, that is, I felt sorry for myself at first. Having cancer may have been my greatest dramatic role. But, thanks to carrying out a meditation given to me through a friend, I was able to change my point of view.[127]

A path of power

Seeking power for selfish purposes eventually has a negative effect. The beauty of eating close to nature is that it gives one power, while at the same time it is unselfish. Why unselfish?

It takes the same number of acres to raise one pound of beef as it takes to raise sixty pounds of soybeans. John Robbins has pointed out that much farmland has been

---

[127]Milo, 1996a, pp. 5-6.

converted to rangeland to satisfy the appetite for meat that has spread globally with American culture. All over the world youth are wearing jeans, forming gangs, listening to western or western-influenced music and eating hamburgers. But rural peoples may be poor, even starving and certainly do not have personal tape recorders let alone personal computers.

People used to believe the Sun revolved around the Earth. Even if we believe that man is the center of everything, we may realize that other creatures know love, have but one mate unto death, feel pain and experience joy. Many younger societies have not yet learned to credit other creatures with intelligent awareness and sensitivity to pain.

When it is necessary for one's survival, even human flesh becomes food. Many little children spontaneously do not want to eat flesh when they understand what it is. If it has a heart and responds to love, do you want to kill it?

When we kill animals out of need, then they are giving their life for us, and we are interconnected with them and they with us. To kill anything wantonly when we do not have a need for it is not right, as any child can tell you.

The cuisine of other parts of the world, when meat is available, involves preparing small amounts of meat scattered in with vegetables or rice. If the people lead the simple life of hunter-gatherers, then everyone eats all the meat all at once, lest it spoil, unless there is enough to preserve it with salt or smoke. But this, unless you live in the Arctic, is a special event.

In the industrialized West, animals are raised the way automobiles are assembled: in animal and poultry factories, and we eat whole hunks and slabs of meat and poultry from our plate. As a result, heart disease is the leading cause of death in American males, and too many people get cancer who might not if they ate differently.

Why does eating plant food confer power?

The power that comes with eating plant food comes from one's alignment with or harmony with Nature, physically, with one's body, and dynamically in terms of the mental and emotional strength that comes with simplicity. This power is also a result of becoming more grounded.

Many westerners, possibly because of a dysfunctional family life,[128] of childhood abuse, possibly because of allergies, pollution or because of eating too many foods which dissipate their energy, are not well *grounded*. This condition contributes to depression or to a distorted or hyper reactive response to physical reality, one which makes it difficult to perceive one's needs. This condition is also discussed by Hermain Aihara in relation to people who have taken drugs[129] for whom, he found, it was particularly difficult to stick to their diet.

Whatever the cause, or whatever one's emotional or mental patterns of behavior may have been, a person who is not fully present physically can become in touch with their body and their needs by eating close to nature, . By being fully present physically, one ceases to be the victim of one's thoughts or at the mercy of one's feelings --- un-anchored, blowing like wisps of cloud in the wind. I know this because at times I used to be that way myself. Working on one's self spiritually helps to keep one on course, and, through introspection, for taking command of one's personality and its evolution.[130]

---

[128]Different published estimates have suggested that between ninety-nine and ninety-five <u>per cent.</u> of American families are dysfunctional.
[129]Aihara, pp.105-106.
[130]Stylianos Atteshlis, Ph.D,, D.D., M.Psy., M.Mcs. "The Esoteric Teachings", *Rev. ed.* 1992, Strovolos Cyprus.

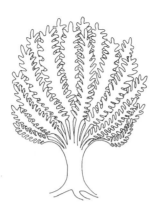

Chapter Ten

Spiritual Help

If we are unable to remove pollutants from our external environment, we can manage them with diet, clean living and exercise. These will help to remove the effects of pollution from our emotional and mental environment as well.

Attitudes toward sickness

The importance of a sick person's attitude in healing has been realized since ancient times. Although ignored in much of the Twentieth Century, respect for the value of one's attitude in healing is again being remembered.

Possibly the greatest healing property of eating close to nature is its effect on one's attitude. The holistic practitioners I consulted: the acupuncturist and the Macrobiotic Dietary Counselors, were not impressed by the fact that I had "cancer". They paid it little mind, taking it for granted that if I ate reasonably well it would go away. The idea of "cancer" was downplayed. There was no fuss about it.

By contrast, when I went to get a check up from a physician every four to six months, I prayed and meditated first in order to prepare myself for the onslaught of his or her attitude to "cancer".

Whether well or sick, we have within us certain feelings and beliefs and above all, a self awareness.

The extreme sensitivity of those who are seriously sick renders them vulnerable to all thoughts coming their way. The attitudes of others are not perceived critically but are accepted immediately as fact by the unconscious mind because a sick person's protective, critical ego barriers are down.

The clinician who encounters a typically withdrawn cancer patient, one who speaks slowly and hesitantly (as from a long way off) is not aware of the intense inward focus the sick person is giving up, even for a few moments, to communicate with him. That is why sick people are withdrawn. As one woman who had a husband and children confided to me: "I don't know if I want to get well; having cancer is such a rush."[131]

Unfortunately, the clinician is unaware of how much devastation his/her words and attitude can cause. Their effect can be fatal if the person with "cancer" does not know how to guard against them or how to reverse the negative programming which can result in severe anxiety.

The most constructive attitude a physician can have is unfailingly to maintain the awareness that a physician does not have divine authority and that anything in our merciful universe is possible. Such is the attitude of the more successful physicians, who by encouraging their patients may inspire them with a will to live when before there was only dread.

Make peace not war?

"There is more than one way to skin a cat", as the old saying goes.

The technical achievements of western medicine have reached almost unimaginable heights while the War on

---

[131]Milo, 1995a.

Cancer admittedly has been lost. But perhaps the Peace with Cancer is being won. Because alternative healing was not institutionalized, there are few extensive studies to prove it.

To get well, once I was eating well, and had learned other lessons that my cancer brought me, all I had to do was to Keep On Keeping On. I kept in mind that Nature heals slowly. Finally I realized, as so many others have, that, although I had "cancer", I was living my life.[132]

I was living my life - but I had "cancer". But I felt well. If I felt well, then I must *be* well. If I had "cancer", then, so what? Evidently it was no big deal. With it or without it, I felt well and was living my life.[133]

I noted that I was healing because some days I had "cancer" and other days I did not. Gradually, the days I had "cancer" grew fewer and farther apart until they ceased to exist.

Keeping On Keeping On was not as easy as I thought it would be. Lying in wait was the enemy that in part had resulted in my getting cancer.

The enemy was the Inner Saboteur in my unconscious mind. Can I define it? The best I can do at this time is: I once again ignored my needs in favor of someone else's wishes, which was followed by deep despair accompanied by a feeling of "what's the use?" This was accompanied by eating a lot of sweets, which soon manifested in a frightening loss of energy and another breast lump.

Over a period of a few months, panicked, I ran around wildly seeking and devising other alternative cures while I continued to lose energy. Then I realized that if I was growing weaker by the day it was not the diet's fault. I had broken my diet. I tightened up on my way of eating and continued my spiritual practices and slowly came into balance again. I was extremely careful to avoid all forms of sugar and had

---

[132]Milo, 1996a.
[133]Milo, 1995a.

night sweats for a month. Then I was back on track and able to fulfill some of my own wishes..

Our friend, Anxiety

Anxiety is the most devastating part of having cancer. It may come on well before we are diagnosed and stays with us until the disease slowly fades away or until we realize that having cancer has a point and a purpose in our life, which has been served. It is our friend because it guides us. If we can manage our anxiety, we can do anything.

I prayed and meditated three times a day to control my anxiety, and also when and if something caused me to feel anxious. The particular meditations I carried out and the holistic measures I followed are in a pamphlet which is a workbook in outline form.[134]

A second very important thing I did was to say, "Yes, I want to live', but I did not say or allow myself to think "I *have* to live", because it is rare that we as humans, are at one with our Soul's intentions and can decide when our lives will end and then depart. Rarely can we apprehend the contents of our unconscious mind.

Does anyone imagine that the Creator does not love Its Creation? Sustained by the conviction that God is Merciful, I have faith in Divine Order. That is to say, I believe that whatever happens to me is for my best possible good in the long run. So when I did not know if I would live or not, I prayed: *Thy Will be done.* Not my will, *Thy* will. The decision may or may not be ours to make. This was a difficult state of mind for me to achieve. It took work. One cannot compel reverence. But it helps.

The most down to earth approach to anxiety is to cook and eat your food with the realization that everything passes. You live your life and keep on keeping on, knowing that the sound of the waves, of wind in the trees, is like our heart beating or our lungs breathing. We are all part of the

---

[134]Milo, 1996a.

same Process, the same rhythm, now and in the worlds beyond place-time in which we also exist. We do not create the Process; It gives us to our Selves.

As soon as I noticed I was improving, I had to face a scarey question. It hit me like a thunderbolt. It was: What will I do without my cancer? This question caused me more anxiety. After thinking about it, I realized that there was no way out. If I wanted to live, I would have to be myself and would have to continue being myself even though I was fairly convinced that nobody would want me or anything I had to offer.

Attitudes to the world

Persons who develop cancer, like me, may not have understood "how life works." In a nutshell, I think that is because we may label other people's wants as 'needs' and our own needs as 'wants'. We do not express even to ourselves, our needs or our wants. Such a stance may be in part due to present and/or previous life programming and habits, and to the "rush" which makes one's inner life so interesting.[135]

Recovery from cancer means reinvolvement with the world, reinvolvement with other people, reinvolvement with exterior existence, and not turning away from it. Yet it need not mean becoming worldly, becoming within as the world is without. We can choose to be "in the world but not of it."

How do we return to being in the world?

Typically, a person who gets cancer does not want to ask anyone for help.[136] Neither did I. I wanted to be self sufficient. But, caught in a double bind, I also wanted to live. I needed information and the help that I knew certain friends could give me.

I endured a certain amount of torment until I gathered up my courage, for I was very afraid of being rejected, and

---

[135]Milo, 1995a.

asked for the help I needed. I was pleasantly surprised at how warm my friends were and at how eager they were to be of help. I began to learn that, unlike what I had thought, people do care; people want to help[137] and that self expression is good.

Could I have thought that people did not care because I myself was not caring? I did care but was doing nothing about it because I thought no one wanted what I had to offer. So, at a friend's urging, I volunteered to teach stress reduction methods in our local prison.

Some of the people in prison were appreciative, not only of what I had to offer but of my caring to be there, and I in turn appreciated their company and what they had to offer: their caring. One man begged me to listen to him and to follow his advice which I did, advice which was based on the experience with radiation treatments of his deceased sister. I shall always remember with love and highest admiration each of those gentlemen. Society does not know their Soul's intent which, above any other reason, sent them to prison.

An attitude toward "cancer"

It was the best thing that ever happened to me. I was so surprised to make this discovery, even before I was well, that I asked other persons with cancer who did not yet know if they would recover, if cancer was not the best thing that had happened to them. After a moment of shock came a smile, and the answer was always: *Yes.*[138] [139] Even my old friend Bill, when near to being overcome with AIDS, responded: "Positively! Decisively, yes! *It is the best thing that happened to me.* " And so it is with any great misfortune.

---

[136]Temoshok and Dreher, *Op. cit.*
[137]Milo, 1995a.
[138]Milo, 1995a
[139]Kushi, 1991, pp. 159-60.

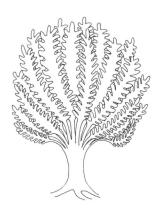

Epilog
Nearly Twenty Years After

Time makes many things clearer, which is why I am adding on this section, which deals mainly with Denial.

I'm not giving much time to the quirks in human nature—in mine and in nearly everyone else's!—which may lead a person with cancer further from health.

One can never say that John or Laura are not getting well because they have failed to take responsibility for their sickness or because they may use their sickness as a bludgeon to exact revenge, deference and service out of everyone around them. Cancer can set one free, as many have discovered, even without knowing the outcome of their illness.

No experience in life, not even cancer or AIDS, is wasted. Sometimes, people cannot help what happens to them—although they can do something about it.

What promoted healing in me was to realize that my sickness was an in-house matter. The drama of my dying or my recovery actually involved only myself, no matter who might be touched or upset by it.

Before I realized this fact, my focus was not on the realness of my living or my dying but on the tragedy of my condition and, unconsciously, on the suffering it might possibly inflict on those dear to me to whom I had never expressed any anger. Mainly, this behavior

1. served as a way to deny my actual, frightening condition. I was focussed on my role as a person with cancer, not on my condition. Fear can easily push one into shifting one's focus.

2. is symptomatic of the repression—even to oneself —of one's feelings, even to the extent that one feels that there is nothing to live for.

That is why Dr. Hamer's[140] identification of the long term role of the double bind situation as a childhood antecedent to cancer rang true to me. The emotional conflicts or wounds which he found to occur five to eight years before diagnosis and again, roughly within six months of diagnosis, again would seem to place one in a repeated double bind so that one's existence seems hopeless and one gives up on it.

I was unaware of my anger when I had "cancer." Yet it served me well because when I had "cancer," my anger became focused. I was so angry that I insisted on doing everything "My Way". Thereby, with invaluable help—to which I was open and even had asked for!—from my friends, I healed.[141]

To say "I did it my way" was healing because I no longer was able or willing to face the world on any other terms.[142] In this way, I recovered lost personal barriers and compensated for my unresolved rage at having been seen, I believed, not as a person but as a role. Unfortunately, this is how many of us learn to relate to each other: as roles rather than as people.

I was saved from the danger of denial by a meditation given me by a friend of friends who said I must go "inside", contact the cancer cells and apologize to them for disrupting their life.[143] A valued friend's comment was:

---

[140]Hamer

[141]Milo, *unpublished manuscript.*

[142]As a friend with breast cancer recently expressed it: "No more Mrs. Nice Guy".

[143]Milo, 1996a.

"Apologize?? That's hard to swallow. Should we apologize to other mass murderers?"

Yes, it was hard to swallow, all right. But cancer, the "out-of-sync" cells within our bodies, is not a mass murderer. The mass murderer is the polluted lifestyle: physical, emotional, mental, and spiritual—they are all linked together—which insults and eventually may corrupt our perfect DNA. Cancer is an ancient disease and the human spirit has faced challenges in every era.

The meditation given me by a friend of friends was so hard to swallow that it took me three days to overcome my anger to the point that I was willing to carry it out. What astonished me about the exercise was that it forced me to take responsibility for my sickness which gave me power over it. What was possibly most important was that it reestablished the integrity of my body and my at-one-ment with all of it, down to the last sick cell which, instead of being a hated enemy became a trusted friend.[144]

Being saved from denial meant that I had to live, for months, in full awareness of how fragile was my grip on earthly existence. I was able to deal with the fear and anxiety generated by my physical condition—since medication did not fit with my lifestyle—through applying the meditations and prayers that already had been the focus of my life for some years. Gradually, my anxiety eased somewhat as eating close to nature improved my physical condition. Eventually it left and I considered myself "cured."

In the Poem, "The Voyage to Ithaca" by the Alexandrian Greek poet, Constantine Cavafy, the voyage is a metaphor for our existence. The wise hero, Odysseus's, voyage home after the Trojan War, not his arrival there, emerges as the point of his life.

Without counting on a "sure thing", without knowing if I would be "cured", I lived and still live my life on a daily basis. Because I was living my life, it gradually ceased to

---

[144]Milo, 1995a.

matter if I had "cancer".

It has now been eighteen years since I received a diagnosis of cancer. It showed me that whatever the course of our existence, we will progress. Through our voyage, we will evolve until our joy is complete.

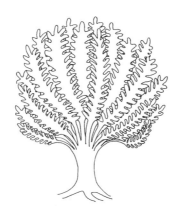

Bibliography

Aihara, Herman. "Acid and Alkaline," George Ohsawa Macrobiotic Foundation, 1986 (first edition 1971) Oroville CA.

_____, "How To Overcome Fear," audio cassette #230, 1996, Kushi Institute.

Asistent, Niro Markoff. Why I survive AIDS. *New Age Magazine*, October, 1991 p. 41. Adapted from 1991: "Why I Survive AIDS," Simon & Schuster/Fireside.

Atteshlis, Stylianos, Ph.d,, D.D., M.Psy., M.Mcs. "The Esoteric Teachings," *Rev. ed.* 1992, Nicosia.

_____, General Lecture Series, Strovolos, Cyprus: selected lectures, 1988-1994.

_____, On the Etheric Double (for Psycho-therapists), *General Lecture*, Feb. 7, 1991, (audio cassette) Nicosia.

Babbitt, Elwood. Arlington Street Church lectures, Boston, 1975-76.

Barnard, M.D., Neal. "Food For Life: How the New Four Food Groups Can Save Your Life," 1993. Crown, NY. Originally published by Harmony Books, 1993, New York.

Bird, Christopher, Gaston Naessens' Symposium on Somatidian Orthobiology: a Beachhead Established, *in The Townsend Letter for Doctors*, October 1991, pp. 797-805.

_____,Progress in Getting the Medical Profession to Focus on the Study of Geopathic Zones and their Effect on Health, *The American Dowser*, 24 (4): 6-13. November 1985.

Brandle E., Sieberth H.G., Hautmann R.E. Effect of dietary protein intake on the renal function in healthy subjects. *Eur. J. Clin. Nutr.*, Nov. 1996 50(11): 734-740.

Brandt, Dr. Johanna. "How to Conquer Cancer, Naturally," 1989 Tree of Life Publications, Palm Springs CA. First published 1929 with original title: "The Grape Cure".

Breuss, Rudolph, "The Breuss Cancer Cure," 1995, *alive* books, Burnaby BC.

Brodeur, Paul, "Currents of Death," 1989. Simon and Schuster

_____, "The Great Powerline Cover-Up," 1993, Little. Brown and Co.

Campbell, T. Colin, quoted in Study: Meat in diet increases disease risk. *The Boston Herald,* May 9,1990, p. 26. This article is a pre-publication summary of data from the 1990 Cornell Study on diet and disease.

Clark, Hulda Regehr, Ph.D.,N.D., "The Cure For All Cancers", 1993, ProMotion Publishing, SanDiego.

Cope, Oliver M.D., "The Breast," 1974, Little Brown.

Davis, Jaquie, "Cancer Winner," 1977, Pacific Press, Pierce City MO.

William Dufty, "Sugar Blues," 1993, Warner Books (1976 reissue).

Epstein, S.S. The Chemical Jungle: Today's Beef Industry. *Int. J. Health Serv.* 1990, 20 (2): 277-280.

East West Foundation with Ann Fawcett and Cynthia Smith, "Cancer-Free: 30 Who Triumphed Over Cancer Naturally," 1991, Japan Publications Inc.

Friend, Sun City, Arizona; 1997, personal communication

Goldberg, Burton, "Alternative Medicine Guide to Women's Health 2," 1998, Future Medicine Publishing, Inc. Tiburon CA.

Gorman, Caroline, "Less Toxic Living," 1993 sixth edition, Environmental Health Center, 8345 Walnut Hill Lane, Dallas TX 75231.

Graeub, Ralph, with *Introduction* by Dr. Ernest Sternglass, "The Petkau Effect," 1992, Four Walls Eight Windows, New York. Translated from the German by Phil Hill. Revised English edition of 1990: "Der Petkau-Effekt," Zytglogge Verlag, Bern.

Gurney J.G., Davis S., Severson R.K., Fang J.Y., Ross J.A., Robison LL., Trends in cancer incidence among children in the U.S. *Cancer*, Aug. 1, 1996, 78(3): 532-541.

Hamer, Dr. Med. Ryke Geerd, "Krebs, der Krankheit das Seele," 1987, Verlag Amici di Dirk, Koln: Gesellschaft Med. Schriften.

Jensen, Bernard, D.C., "Iridology Simplified," 1980, Dr. Bernard Jensen, 24360 Old Wagon Rd., Escondido CA 92027.

Karp, Harvey M.D., quoted in *The Green Guide,* June 1, 1998, (54/55), p.2.

Kerstetter J.E.,Caseria D.M., Mitnick M.E., Ellison A.F., Gay L.F., Liskov T.A., Carpenter T.O. and Insogna K.L. Increased circulating concentrations of parathyroid hormone in healthy young women consuming a protein-restricted diet. *Am. J. Clin. Nutr.* Nov., 1997 66(5): 1188-1196.

Klahr, S., Is there still a role for a diet very low in protein, with or without supplements, in the management of patients wth endstage renal failure? *Curr. Opin. Nephrol. Hypertens.* July, 1996, 5(4):384-387.

Kroeger, Rev. Hanna, Ms.D. "Free your body of tumors and cysts," 1997, Hanna Kroeger Publications.

Kushi, Michio, "Standard Macrobiotic Diet," 1996. One Peaceful World Press, Becket MA

_____, "How to See Your Health: Book of Oriental Diagnosis," 1980, Japan Publications, Inc., New York and Tokyo.

_____ with Edward Esko, "The Macrobiotic Approach to Cancer," 1991, Avery, Garden City NY.

_____ and Martha C. Cotrell, M.D. with Mark N. Mead, "AIDS, Macrobiotics and Natural Immunity," 1990, Japan Publications, Inc.

_____ and Aveline Kushi, "Macrobiotic Diet," Edited by Alex Jack. 1985, Japan Publications, Inc.

Lemonick, Michael D., What's wrong with our sperm? *Time Magazine*, March 18, 1996,: 78-79.

LeShan, Lawrence "Cancer as a Turning Point," Plume, 1990.

Levels of smog raising alarm, *USA Today*, June 24,1998, p.5D.

Levey, A.S., Adler S., Caggiula, A.W., England B.K., Greene T., Hunsicker L.H., Kusick J.W., Rogers N.L.and Teschan P.E.:L Effects of Dietary Protein Restriction on the Progression of Advanced Renal Disease in the Modification of Diet in Renal Disease Study. *Am. J. Kidney Dis.* May 1996, 27 (5): 652-663.

Livingston, Virginia, M.D., "The Conquest of Cancer," Livingston Foundation Medical Center, San Diego.

Mackenzie H.S., Brenner B.M. Current strategies for retarding progression of renal disease. *Am. J. Kidney Dis.,* Jan. 1998 31(1): 161-170.

Milo, Antonia G., "A Double Axe: Cancer and the Mind," 1996a. Balanced Way, Fernandina FL.

_____, Further Aspects of Decision Making in Persons with Cancer or AIDS. *Phoenix Rising IV: Proc. Int. Conf. On the Study of Shamanism and Alt. Modes of Healing,* 1996b: 106-109.

_____, lecture presented at the 12th International Conference on the Study ofShamanism, 1995a, audio cassette, Balanced Way.

_____, Bridging Worlds: Decision Making of Indiviudals with Cancer or AIDS. Paper derived from lecture, in *Proc. Int. Conf. On the Study of Shamanism and Alt. Modes of Healing,* 1995b: 272-274.

_____, *manuscript in preparation.*

Muramoto, Noboru,"Natural Immunity: Insights on Diet and AIDS," 1988. George Ohsawa Macrobiotic Foundation, Oroville.

Northrup, Christiane, M.D., "Women's Bodies, Women's Wisdom," 1994, Ballantine

Ohsawa, George, "Macrobiotics - the Way of Healing," 1981. George Ohsawa Foundation Press, Oroville CA.

Okun, M. and Edelstein, L., The Cell and the Organism: the Role of Subdivisional Cell Replication in the Development and Maintenance of a Multicellular Organism. *Cell Biology International* 1995, 19 (10): 851-877.

Peters C., Lotzerich H., Niemeier K.,Schule K, Uhlenbruck G., Influence of a moderate exercise training on natural killer cytotoxicity and personality traits in cancer patients. *Anticancer Res.* May,1994, 14 (3A): 1033-1036.

Rampa, Teusday Lobsang, "Doctor From Lhasa," 1980, Corgi.

Physicians Committee for Responsible Medicine, P.O. Box 6322, Washington DC 20015. *PCRM Update*, May-June 1991.

Randolph, Bonnie, Return to Life: How I Defied My Doctor and Survived Ovarian Cancer, *EastWest Journal*, November/December, 1991.

Read, Anne, Carol Ilstrup and Margaret Gammon under the editorship of Hugh Lynn Cayce, "Edgar Cayce on Diet and Health," 1969, Warner Books.

Robbins, John, "May All Be Fed: Diet for a New World," 1992, William Morrow NY.

Rodale, J., 1970: "Happy People Rarely Get Cancer," Rodale Press Inc., Emmaus PA.

Sheldrake, Rupert, Ph.D., "A New Science of Life: the Hypothesis of Morphic Resonance," Tarcher 1982.

Simonton, O. Carl, Stephanie Matthews-Simonton and James L. Creighton, "Getting Well Again: a Step By Step, Self Help Guide To Overcoming Cancer For Patients and Their Families," 1978, Bantam.

Stapleton, Ruth Carter "The Experience of Inner Healing," 1977, World Books,

Sternglass, Ernest, with *Introduction* by George Wald, "Secret Fallout," 1981, McGraw-Hill paperback edition, an expanded version of "Low-Level Radiation" first published in 1972 by Ballantine Books.

Stone, Christopher, First Geopathic Congress on Geopathic Stress in Cyprus, 1997, in *The American Dowser* 38 (1):32, Winter, 1998.

Alex Tannous, Dr. Div.,*Creative Living,* c.e.u. courses, 1983, 1984, University of Southern Maine School of Nursing.

Valentine, Tom, Kombucha, a Fermented Beverage With Real 'Zing' In It!, *Search For Health* ! (6), July/Aug. 1993 pp. 1-14.

Walser, M., Effects of a supplemented very low protein diet in predialysis patients on the serum albumin level, proteinuria, and subsequent survival on dialysis. *Miner. Electrolyte Metab.*1998 24(1): 64-71.

Weil, Andrew, M.D.,"Spontaneous Healing," 1995, Fawcett Columbine.

Weiss, Brian, M.D. "Through Time Into Healing," Simon and Schuster, 1992. Chapter 4: *Healing the Body by Healing the Mind*, pp. 56-76.

Wigmore, Ann, "The Wheatgrass Diet," 1985, Avery .

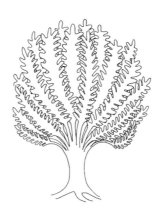

Appendix

Spaghetti

Spaghetti is noodles. Noodles are common food, worldwide, except, perhaps, in the very northerly meat-and-potatoes climates where grain is hard to grow. Most of us in the United States eats spaghetti from time to time, especially when we are in a hurry but not buying junk food. By making just a few changes in what you do with the spaghetti, you can take a step to better health.

One way to begin is to recognize that there are many kinds of spaghetti. The ones we like are made of *durum* or spelt wheat, wheat that has been around a long time and has fewer chromosomes. Is it a kinder, gentler wheat? Hard to say. But a basic principle of the natural, "macrobiotic" diet which helped me to cure my breast cancer, is to eat low on the evolutionary tree. That means eating foods that have been around the longest, such as seaweeds, beans and legumes, vegetables, and grains: grains that are closest to nature with a gene pool that has been relatively unaffected by human manipulation or selection over generations.

There is spaghetti made of artichoke for people with wheat allergies, and in the Orient, spaghetti - they are flat like noodles, and made without eggs - from wheat, brown rice, and buckwheat.

Should you be a person with cancer working to heal yourself naturally, including the "macrobiotic" diet I used, you will most likely be eating two kinds of whole grain every day, and once a day at least, one bowl of brown rice, and when you want a snack, snacking on brown rice. But it can be a pleasant change to have noodles once or twice a week if your macrobiotic counsellor says it is appropriate for your physical condition. If so, you may follow all the suggestions below except for tomatoes.

Tomatoes and all nightshades, including eggplants, peppers and potatoes are avoided when healing oneself. Otherwise, they are generally avoided unless you live in a hot, *"yang"* climate, for these nightshade vegetables are very *"yin,"* or expanding and cooling, and in addition are prone to pulling up chemical toxins out of the earth.

Two pots, or one pot plus one fry pan.
cutting board
straight-blade knife.

1. Heat water for boiling spaghetti. High flame.

2. Enough olive oil or corn oil to half-cover bottom of fry pan or second pot (thick bottom). When I had cancer, I was told to avoid all oil "for now." You can saute the vegetables in water and it's very nice. I often use just water to saute vegetables. Near the end of cooking, I add a little fine quality soy sauce (no MSG!) and stir it in. By using soy sauce, I do not need grated cheese for flavoring. This is useful to know if your health can be improved by avoiding all dairy products, as I (usually) do.

Options. Choose one or more:
Onions
Leeks

Mushrooms
Spaghetti sauce
Tomatoes

With chopping knife and cutting board, chop onions, one or two, and (medium flame) sizzle in olive oil or corn oil till transparent or they start to turn brown. Don't forget to stir them or turn them. If you add more options, you may add more oil.

Same with mushrooms.

Same with tofu, sliced 1/4 - ½ inch thick. Cut one or two of these slabs into smaller squares if you like and save the rest in a bowl of fresh water in frig. (Cover bowl).

Chop a pile of fresh of fresh parsley after rinsing it and shaking off excess water.

Do not fry but put to one side for later.

Open container of spaghetti sauce (Ragu is good) and heat in pan or second pot, with or without options. While sauce is heating, put spaghetti in boiling water. Boil spaghetti for about three minutes. Drain by dumping into a colander, or pour off water.

Some people like to run their drained spaghetti under cold water to stop it from cooking more. The next step is to put the semi-cold spaghetti on a plate and pour the sauce over it. But...there is another way: just drain the spaghetti and dump it into the pot with the sauce and options and mix together.

Serve. Add other options: fresh chopped parsley
Grated Parmesan cheese

Spaghetti is also very nice when served with options but no spaghetti sauce. Or you may wish to put your own chopped fresh tomatoes in with the options if you have a garden.

As you may have noted, steps 2 and 3 are optional. You may substitute water sauteing instead, if you want to take in very little fat.

For flavoring in water sauteing, we recommend investing in a very good soy sauce without preservatives, MSG (monosodium glutamate) or other additives.

Water sauteing:

Have the vegetables chopped first. Suggested vegetables are carrots, onion, cabbage, leeks, mushrooms, even bok choy and Chinese cabbage- they are an acquired taste. Put the carrots in first with water to cover the bottom of the pan. Stir them from time to time and add a little water as necessary. When the carrots seem to be soft, add the chopped onions, then the cabbage, adding small amounts of water as needed. When nearly cooked, dribble in soy sauce to taste but very little as it is salty. Mushrooms or tofu chunks are options as is chopped parsley to put on top.
I also like to water saute with kale, collards, or turnip greens, sometimes with onions, sometimes without.

Water sauteed vegetables are good with spaghetti but I prefer them with brown rice.

Brown rice

Sick or healthy, at least half one's diet can be grains. Much of this can be a bowl of brown rice eaten daily. In winter in the North it is good to use short grain brown rice cooked in a pressure cooker with a small pinch of salt. This will help to keep a person warm.

In Florida winters, for example, medium grain brown rice is better for the sick who do not easily digest brown rice and boiled, not pressure cooked.

In hot weather, long grain brown rice or basmati rice or even white rice or a mix of white and brown rice is better because this rice, more expanded in form (longer rather than rounder) is more *yin*, or cooling.

For the sick who do not easily digest brown rice, it can be made into a cream by pressure cooking or boiling with a lot of water and a little salt for a very long time. Serve with a little weak miso soup. Sages have lived on nothing but brown rice and miso soup.

How to boil rice:

People learn how to cook their rice just right after about two weeks of trial and error.

1. Wash rice. This is important. Pour off floating grains, dust, insect eggs? Etc.

2. Add about one and a half times as much water as rice. Throw in a small pinch of salt unless the weather is very hot. It is important to have a flame tamer if you are cooking with gas. Comment about electric and microwave cooking: it tends to zap the food (cooking it by exploding it rather than by heating it).

Bring to a boil on medium or medium-high flame and cook with lid slightly off the pot until the water is gone and there are little wells or holes all over the surface of the rice, but before you smell it burning. Put clean dish towel over pot, beneath lid, remove from flame and let it steam until you are ready to eat it.

3. Take the dish towel away if you refrigerate the rice, but the best way to save it is in a bowl, on the counter, with cheesecloth or dish towel over the top. It will keep in this way up to three days. Longer is not good. When food is stale, even though still edible and without mold, it drags a person down instead of being energizing.

4. There are many things to put on top of rice besides oleo or butter or grease. If you wish to avoid animal fat because you have a heart problem, or wish simply to avoid fat because you may have cancer or need to lose weight, consider chopped green onions, chopped parsley, a Japanese flavoring called "*gomashio*", also known as 'sesame salt', sunflower seeds, or roasted pumpkin seeds- all seeds, even peanuts if they appear to be freshly roasted, in moderation, just enough for flavor, for a low fat diet.

The sesame salt complements the protein in the rice and, used sparingly, is delicious. We recommend using it sparingly because, unless you make your own, the proportion of salt is rather high for regular use, especially in warm weather.

Water sauteed vegetables are very good to put with the rice. Or, such vegetables can be sauteed in a little oil, or in a little oil first then adding water to keep the vegetables from sticking. That makes it very low fat.

Warning, or Healthy Kitchen Practices: No aluminum pots.

Wash your vegetables. Particularly greens.

An easy way to get rid of pesticides is to put a splash or clorox in the pot or sink you wash veggies in. Let vegetables soak for ten minutes. Then change the water and let soak ten more minutes. Or buy "Clean Greens" at a health store and follow instructions to wash vegetables.

Back to spaghetti #1:
You may also think of spaghetti as a soup.

A pasta soup is very nice as an evening meal, perhaps with some cornbread or by itself.

Digression on sweets:
I like to chase my pasta soup with corn tortillas (no fat) warmed in an iron skillet, spread with a little tahini, a.k.a. 'sesame butter'. It is a much lighter butter than peanut

butter which I also use on occasion for variety. With it I apply some jam or jelly, the kind sweetened with fruit (pear or grape) juice concentrate rather than with sugar. The sugar content is usually 5%. I buy Sorrell Ridge, which is expensive, but use it sparingly and with it avoid artificial sweeteners which do not help the LIVER. I also have tortillas or whole wheat pita like this for breakfast ... unless I (occasionally) go out.

Good news! Is the nonsugar but powerful sweetener "stevia". Made from the leaves of a tropical tree, it looks like sugar and has a slightly bitter flavor. It is wonderful in lemonade. I think good jams and jelly could be made with it.

Some artificial sweeteners are associated with the development of brain tumors (as is the excessive use of electric blankets!).

Please read the labels on carbonated soft drinks. Do you recognize the ingredients? Ginger ale or some coke is good for an upset stomach, but a carpet tack left overnight in a bottle of coke will dissolve. Most soft drinks have a chemical or sucrose based appeal. I never drink them.

If you have been taking too many sweets, chocolate, etc., try appeasing the sweet tooth with "yinnie" (brown rice syrup) on toast. Of course, eating *yang* foods such as meat, poultry, fertilized eggs, caviar and game fish frequently will result in cravings not only for sweets but for coffee, alcohol, and possibly, dairy products and even drugs. If your body can tolerate such extremes of *yang* and *yin* as these, well and good. May you enjoy them! But...your body will be more stressed, in time, than if you avoided eating regularly food that is at extremes of *yang* or *yin*.

Digression on baked goods:

Why would I have tortillas for breakfast instead of toast?

Answer: they taste good. But, also, according to Oriental medicine, baked goods are not good for the heart. If you stop to consider it, most of what many of us eat are in fact, baked goods. Incidentally, corn and corn products are good for the heart. If baked goods are minimized at breakfast by eating cereals, grits or, traditionally Oriental style, brown rice with sesame salt and a little miso soup, it is easy to not eat too many, **unless** a person is extremely fond of baked snacks, to wit: Frito, Cheetos, crackers, cookies, etc. Unfortunately, many of these can be ingested as snacks. Suggested replacements are: tortillas (not the fried chips if one wants low fat):

> Green onions
> Radishes
> Carrot sticks
> Occasionally olives
> A few dried raisins or other dried fruits - limited
>> amount
> Sunflower seeds (unsalted)
> Pumpkin seeds (unsalted or lightly salted)
> Soy cheeses
> Baked tofu pieces (pre-cooked; taste like
>> smoky cheese or bologna).

Back to spaghetti #2:

For a nice spaghetti soup:

½ pot of water (about a pint and a half, or 3/4 of a quart) on a flame tamer, flame medium or medium high.

Drop in a little piece of seaweed (wakame).

All of the following are options.

Cut a few slices of ginger

Cut a few slices of hot pepper.

Shave a carrot (like whittling a stick) or chop into chunks.

Peel and slice 2 ½ inch thick slices of butternut squash, and cut into chunks.

When the water is boiling but not too fast add any or

all the above. Then:

Cut one small potato in small chunks and add. While
          the above are cooking, cut and add as you go:
one onion cut in eighths or ½ a leek,
3-6 collard, turnip or kale leaves, washed, split down
          the middle and chopped, including stems.
½ a box of spaghetti, broken into thirds. After
          you add the spaghetti, stir the soup from time
          to time while you chop.
1 leaf of plain or Chinese cabbage, split and
          chopped.
4-6 brown mushrooms, washed with tops of stems cut
          off, and halved.

Because other items have been cooking as you go,
you need to continue cooking this only one, perhaps two
more minutes more before it's ready. So have on hand
some good quality soy sauce (no preservatives) and add
some (about 2 tablespoons?). And, if desired, add about the
same amount of *mirin* (Japanese cooking wine) which goes
beautifully with the vegetables and soy sauce. Allow to
blend in the last half minute of cooking.

When I had cancer I avoided potato and *mirin* or
cooking wine, or any alcohol whatever. (Eventually, I sometimes drank beer when eating fish. The idea is: the *yin*,
expanding, relaxing alcoholic drink balances the *yang*,
contracting, condensed energy of the fish). Because I ate
whole grains at nearly every meal, I would have made this
soup with leftover rice, or with whole millet, possibly with
barley. But for some reason I dislike barley in soup. I prefer
to eat barley hot, cooked mixed in with brown rice, or at
room temperature as a salad.

Unless it is a northern midwinter, I try to maintain a
ratio of 3 green vegetables for every root vegetable.

Recipe for delicious barley salad:

Options:
red, yellow or green bell pepper
scallions
parsley
cilantro
small, black olives, possibly oil-cured.
vine-ripened tomato (Edgar Cayce says that tomatoes which are not vine-ripened are very toxic and should only be eaten cooked).
Corn kernels

If you are a purist -I'm not!, blanch (dunk in boiling water) and peel a red, yellow and/or green pepper. Cut in thin slivers and chop them fine. Chop everything else except the olives and corn, and mix everything in with the barley. Add olive oil in moderation and vinegar to taste. You might consider trying Oriental vinegars: brown rice vinegar and my favorite: umeboshi vinegar, made from pickled salted plums. You can find these in a health food store.

If the barley is lukewarm when you mix in the ingredients, you can turn the bowl it is stored in upside down to serve and it will come out very nicely molded and keep its shape. It is a nice party dish for summer, even for a party of 1. I like to garnish it with watercress or parsley. Of course I eat the garnish. "Waste not, want not", and it is so nourishing. How many people suspect that watercress contains generous amounts of both iron and calcium?

Notes about brown rice:

Grain, the seeds of grasses, is the "staff of life."
Wheat and rye are the staff of life in northern and western countries. Corn was the staff of life in North

America. Rice is the staff of life in the Far East. Millet, oats, buckwheat and barley are also frequently eaten in different places. These grains come in several varieties. The most balanced of the grains is rice.

By "balanced", we mean that rice falls in the mid range of *yang* and *yin.* For this reason, it is a calming food. Eating it has a calming effect.

When we speak of rice we are referring to the unrefined, brown rice which keeps all its nutrients. There are many kinds of rice and rices of all colors, but I use the short grain, long grain and medium grain, organically grown brown rice. I eat a bowl of it nearly every day, just as I used to do when I had cancer, only then I often ate two bowls a day or used it as a snack.

The balanced quality of brown rice makes it a wonderful food for the sick because it demands little accommodation by the body to an extreme of *yang,* such as meat, poultry or fish, or even a *yang* grain like buckwheat, or to an extreme of *yin,* such as to dairy products, sugars, soft drinks and non-regional fruit out of season.

The most *yang,* or short grain brown rice is best eaten in most *yin,* or cold, damp climate. Eaten in a warm climate, it will make a person feel too hot. But if a person is very *yin:* sick, weak or debilitated or suffering from a *yin* (peripheral) type of cancer such as of the skin or the breast, eating short grain brown rice can be helpful. Because the macrobiotic way of eating does not go to extremes, but eats regionally and seasonally, it is best to eat the variety of rice that will grow in the kind of climate in which you are living.

In New England, short grain brown rice is nice for winter and medium grain for summer. Sixty per cent of the diet can be whole grains. But in Florida, for example, medium grain brown rice is good for winter with long grain brown rice, or even some white rice and much less rice, or whole grain in general, is good for summer.

Cooking methods are important in connection with

climate and the physical condition of a person. The addition of salt, heat, and pressure through pressure cooking renders food more *yang:* more contracting, more heating, more energizing. Using no pressure, less salt, and less heat or more water, as in boiling or steaming lightly, is a more *yin* way of preparing food which is still much more *yang* than eating raw food or a diet of raw fruit.

Hominy, or corn grits, is wonderful for the summer Southern USA and all year round. Yellow corn grits are cooked as *polenta* in Italy and served with tomato sauce and grated cheese like spaghetti. Or they can be served with water sauteed or oil and water sauteed vegetables to which a little soy sauce has been added.

Corn which is not organically grown and carefully treated can develop mold called *aflatoxins* (as can peanuts) which can promote the development of cancer. So I prefer to eat organically grown grits and organically grown corn, when I can.

A little sea salt added to grain before cooking makes it more digestible. If a person is sick and weak and is having trouble digesting food, one can prepare for them, as for babies, a brown rice cream. This is done by pressure cooking the brown rice - or boiling, for along time until it becomes creamy. A small amount served with a little sesame salt on top and a small cup of miso soup with a little seaweed in it should be tolerated and absorbed well.

Chopped parsley or watercress is always an option on top of soup. Parsley is especially helpful in breaking up kidney stones and in cleaning kidneys.

Soy sauce and *miso*

Why use Japanese ingredients like soy sauce and mirin, which is wine made from rice?

Answer: By royal edict, in order to avoid a plague,

Japan was pisco-vegetarian from 675 AD until the mid-Nineteenth Century when Western (American) traders began to persuade them to eat meat. In the course of twelve hundred years, they developed two main ingredients which add a meatier-than-meaty flavor to soups, stews, and other vegetable dishes. The first of these is soy sauce.

A good quality soy sauce can be found in a health food store and is quite different from that found in the supermarket, as well as being more expensive. The flavor in the better soy cause comes from the natural ingredients, whereas more commercial brands rely on artificial flavors such as MSG (monosodium glutamate) to which some people are allergic, and which adds a more metallic flavor.

We have mentioned using soy sauce above. It comes in two varieties: *tamari* and *shoyu.* Shoyu is made from sea salt, fermented soybeans, and wheat. Somewhat stronger, but better for persons allergic to wheat, is tamari, which is simply made from fermented soybeans, sea salt and water.

Soy sauce is best added to food near the end of cooking so as to conserve the digestive enzymes in it. When people pour it on top of food after cooking, they tend to add too much, because the flavor has not had time to "marry" with the food, This habit can lead to eating too much salt and eventually, a craving for sweets.

A second great gift from the Far East is *miso.* Miso is fermented soybean paste and comes in many varieties. Some are more *yang* or *yin* than others. A good, middle of the road *miso* for a sick person is made with fermented soybeans, barley and sea salt. It is dark brown. This is called "Mugi miso." It was the only miso I used when I had breast cancer (a *yin* condition; living in New England; a *yin* climate; in the city; a *yang* environment). But in a warm climate, less dense than a city, a light brown or yellow miso makes better eating.

The traditional Japanese breakfast is brown rice with a little sesame salt sprinkled on it, perhaps a bowl of greens (collards, turnips or kale) and a small cup of *miso* soup. When one is sick, all portions should be small. Ideally, all portions should always be small, but vegans, people who eat neither meat, poultry, fish nor dairy products sometimes consume enormous amounts of food.

Because I had to cook my breakfast and the lunch I carried with me to work, this is usually what I did when I got up in the morning: I started pressure cooking three cups of rice on a medium high flame so it would come to pressure quickly and soon be ready. Living further South, I boil the same amount of rice over a medium high flame so that it quickly (in about ten minutes) boils away all the water, leaving little pits or holes in the surface of the rice which I then cover with a dish towel beneath the lid and allow it to steam for twenty minutes or a half hour. This is enough rice to last for two or three days.

Before I start the rice, I have put a piece of *wakame* seaweed the size of a fingernail to soak in one or two cups of water in a pot. When I have started cooking the rice, in the soup pot I put a 2-inch-long piece of daikon, the long Oriental white radish. Over it I set a steamer, and in the steamer I place a carrot, a stalk of broccoli or a quarter of califlower, a leek or an onion, maybe half a turnip. Beneath, I turn the flame medium. Then I go to wash and dress for work.

When I am ready for work I come back to the stove, take the rice off the flame and let the pressure go down, if in a pressure cooker, or place a towel on top to allow steaming if I boiled it. I remove the steamer with vegetables from the soup pot and allow them, to cool. I stir l/2 a teaspoon of miso into the soup pot with the daikon and wakame, cooking on lowered flame for ½ minute longer.

Then I serve myself brown rice, sprinkle a little sesame salt on top of it, and have my miso soup.

This was breakfast. Sometimes I added a few pieces of tofu to my miso soup. When I had cancer I used tempeh instead of tofu because tempeh is less processed and less *yin*.

After breakfast I packed in a flat plastic storage dish a generous serving of brown rice, which I sometimes cooked with a little whole wheat or whole barley, or pre-soaked dried chestnuts, for variety; the vegetables I had steamed (organically grown if possible, the juice from which had enriched my soup) and a pickle or a little sauerkraut for more digestive enzymes. The digestive enzymes are especially important if a person has cancer. Then I sprinkled the whole lightly with sesame salt (I made my own, low-salt variety) and that was my lunch for work. It was certainly healthier than sandwiches of greasy lunch meat or even tuna fish or bacon, lettuce and tomato. The other people at work liked to see me open my lunch box and to imagine eating that fresh-looking food themselves.

Notes on ingredients in *miso* soup

miso: Remember to be moderate! A light salty flavor is what you want -a hint of it, only. Otherwise, you will begin to crave sweets.

wakame seaweed: use lightly and, if you live by the sea, very sparingly.

options: to taste.

daikon: helps remove animal fat deposits from the body.

chopped scallions

tempeh

tofu

greens (kale, collards, turnip)

watercress

shitake mushroom

Pizza

Pizza is bonding agent. The children of people from diverse cultures all like it. It is delicious but very fatty, and with the cheese and tomato topping, rather *yin*, not a great cold-weather dish if you want to feel comfortable and warm.

If you are sick, pizza is something to avoid. I did not eat pizza or even taste it for several years. Even now, I do not send out for pizza. But...I found a way to make pizza that is unbelievable and which my son in law enjoyed so much he opened a bottle of red wine to enjoy with it. The ingredients of this wonderdish are only slightly, subtly different from those in regular pizza.

For the pizza itself, I use a loaf of whole wheat pita bread. I usually buy this at the health food store because in the supermarket, the wholewheat pita has calcium propionate or sodium benzoate or something "to retard spoilage." Out of respect for my liver, I avoid preservatives as well as alcohol.

Digression on alcohol

Yes, it can delicious. Occasionally a little pure wine, without sulfites added to preserve it, without extra sugar added to ferment it, can be a treat and a digestive when eating seafood. Even so, I cut mine in half by adding an equal or greater amount of water. I would as soon do without it.

Wine, being fruit based, evolved more recently than did the grasses of the field which give us not only bread but beer. Beer does not rob energy in the same way that wine does. There are excellent non alcoholic beers which are what I occasionally enjoy. When I had cancer I never had alcohol or beer of any kind.

Why the avoidance of alcohol? It is hard on a toxic person's liver. It is very *yin,* and will make you very *yin* (hung over) if you take too much of it. People who eat meat, poultry, etc., tolerate alcohol better and the alcohol helps them to balance the flesh food they are eating.

Back to pizza

There are several soy mozzarellas on the market as well as one made from brown rice which I have not tried in pizza. The one that works best in pizza is not pure soy but has in it some casein, or milk protein. Somehow the casein promotes perfect, cheesy melting, but is also like glue, sticking tight to the plate like any melted cheese.

Options:

small round onions, cut in half-moon slices (lengthwise)
tomatoes? Cut the same way
mushrooms, brown ones, cut in wedges
leeks, sliced
parsley, chopped fine and saved for pouring over pizza just before eating.

After spreading slabs of soy cheese on pizza and arranging the options you select, drizzle the whole with (cold pressed) virgin? Olive oil and a fine quality soy sauce. Place under the broiler on a medium flame until the cheese melts. Turn up the flame for a moment if you want the food crisp on top.

You can also cook the pizza in a heavy cast iron frying pan with lid, adding a little oil on the bottom to keep the bread from sticking. It is best to use a flame tamer and a medium-low flame.

Add parsley and enjoy!

Seaweeds

These are also referred to as 'sea vegetables'. The idea of eating them at first was repellant. They are fabulous for supplying minerals to a devitalized, malnourished body and for maintaining a healthy one. Consuming them is a sure way to get enough iodine.

As I live by the sea, I eat little seaweed because sea minerals are present in the air I breathe. When I had cancer and was living in Boston, I ate seaweed very often although in small amounts: a half inch of wakame or kombu (kelp) in my miso soup, and 1-3" cooked with about a cup of beans. Beans were always cooked with seaweed which eliminates gas and complements minerals. Seaweed is very important in medicinal cooking.

Nori comes sundried in flat sheets. It is the easiest seaweed to get used to. It is used for wrapping sushi rolls and making rice balls, and can be eaten as a snack. If the sheets of nori you buy have not been toasted, you will have to toast them over the flame on the stove. Its color will change from purple to green.

Arame and hiziki are two mysterious seaweeds which somewhat look like lumpy dried black string. When one has learned to cook them, and appreciate them, they have a unique flavor which is ... delicious. I recommend consulting a macrobiotic cookbook and reading all about seaweeds and how to cook them

Beans

Beans are always or nearly always cooked with seaweed, if one is eating the Japanese version of a natural diet. I never eat beans without adding seaweed also, because the seaweed does something almost indefinable to the texture of the cooked beans which I have never found duplicated in any other way.

Since persons with cancer must ingest *very* little fat, they should eat only beans which have low fat content. Soybeans are out as they are quite fatty. The only soybean product I ate while my cancer was being cured was tempeh two or three times a week, in small amounts. Tempeh, as we have mentioned above, is a cheese-like fermented cake of partly crushed whole soybeans. In my opinion, tempeh can be more delicious if the cake is sliced horizontally before cutting into smaller pieces, to make thinner slabs.

The beans with low fat content that I cooked and ate when I had cancer were lentils, chick-peas (garbanzo beans) and a Japanese bean called an 'aduki'or 'azuki' bean. Azuki beans are small and dark red and said to be especially good for promoting kidney function. These are mainly the beans I eat today. I have added dried baby limas, very occasionally fava beans (found in Middle Eastern grocery stores; they are called "*foul*" and pronounced "fool"), and anasazi beans, grown by the ancient Native Americans of the Southwest. Anasazi beans resemble pinto beans but have more protein and less fat. I make meatless chili with them and have them with rice or in whole wheat pita bread. All these beans except lentils and sometimes azuki beans must be soaked overnight. When I feel like eating beans, have none cooked and little time for cooking, I prepare red lentils which will be cooked in about ten minutes. I love black beans, too but would as soon open a can. These will clog the valve on your pressure cooker.

Although eating fresh food is important, if you are in a rush and find yourself opening a can of beans, you can drizzle olive oil and lemon juice on top, serve with sliced raw onion, and mop up the gravy with bread.

Before I offer three bean recipes, any bean at all can be delicious just boiled and served hot with thick olive oil, lemon juice to taste, half a raw onion and sourdough bread, Greek style. Who could ask for anything more? But this treat is for enjoying after your recovery from what ails you.

Azuki beans
These beans do not need soaking. They will be cooked in about an hour. Soaked, the cooking time will be a

little less.

I put about 2 inches of kombu in a pot of water and let it soften, then add about a cup of beans and cook on medium low flame, covered but with the lid slightly to one side so as not to have overflow, for about an hour or a little longer. To soften the beans, and this works with all varieties, you can "shock" them by letting the cooking water run low and replenishing it by dribbling cold water down the inside of the pot, not directly on the beans. To shock beans once or twice during cooking has a nice effect on their texture.

One can cook azuki beans with different things (while retaining the kombu). You can add a tangerine, skin and all, to the pot. It should be an organically grown tangerine to avoid dye and pesticides. An apple instead of a tangerine has a different effect. One can also cook azuki beans with butternut squash. This has fabulous results. Use twice as much butternut squash as beans. If the squash is not organically grown, peel what you will use. Cut into about 1-inch chunks and put in the pot on top of the beans about 20 minutes before the end of cooking. You can sprinkle a little sea salt on top. When the squash is soft (the azuki beans remain slightly firm) mix them and the pot liquor together and enjoy with brown rice and a nice bowl of greens.

Chickpeas

Soak overnight. The volume will double. Let an inch of kombu soften in the water in which you have soaked one half cup of chickpeas. Add more water and boil from one to two hours. Halfway through the cooking, and maybe near the end also, I add 4 or 5 cloves of garlic cut lengthwise, and rosemary. I try to shock the chickpeas, too. There should be little water left in the pot when beans - any beans - are ready, unless you are making soup.

The chickpeas will be fragrant and very attractive as a snack as well as part of a meal.

If it is summer and I have time, I make hommus with

the chickpeas. This involves mashing them well and adding sea salt, sesame butter (tahini) and lemon juice to taste. Adding crushed garlic or even garlic powder is an option I like, as well as a swirl of olive oil over paprika on top before sopping it up with bread.

Lentils

The humble lentil can be transformed into quite a powerhouse, yielding a very rich and meaty flavor while sitting very lightly in the stomach. In India, even babies are given *dal*, which can made by first browning onions until they are almost black, then adding water and (brown) rice to the pot. Thirty minutes before the rice is cooked, add lentils in one third or a quarter of the amount of rice. Salt to taste. Traditionally, serve with a little yoghurt on top. But we will have none of this here! Dal is very good without yoghurt too.

For cooking lentils or lentil soup, I soften an inch or kombu or wakame in four times as much water by volume as lentils. Put the lentils in and boil on medium flame, partly covered. You may add the following options:

shitake mushrooms. If you want to add these, soak them in advance unless they are fresh. I like the dried ones more in soup; they are more pungent.

onions, small, round, organically grown. They will be *hot*! I halve them or cook them whole. If I am cooking onions with lentils, I also add to the pot 2 or 3 cloves for a richer, deeper, more rounded flavor.

carrots, 1 or 2, organically grown, in one-inch chunks.

miso. When the lentils are cooked, turn the flame to low and mash one or two tablespoons of mugi miso against the side of the pot, mixing it in with the lentils. Keep sampling it so as not to put in too much miso and make the soup too salty. Turn off flame.

parsley. Chop while the lentils are boiling. Throw as
much as you like on top.

Serve this dish as a soup if it is fairly liquid, or as
beans with or over brown rice.

If this dish starts out being soupy, the portion you
save overnight will soak up a lot of liquid and be
much drier the next day.

A Lebanese friend sautes a chopped leek in a little
olive oil, then adds water and a cup of red lentils. They
cook in ten minutes. She adds olive oil, beats until smooth,
and adds fresh lemon juice to taste, which turns the mixture
a creamy white. Add sea salt and pepper to taste. The
pepper and oil might be best left out if you are seriously
sick.

Greens

I will here deal with the greens, excluding salad and
cabbage, that I ate when I had cancer. I still eat them twice
or more a week and love them. There is nothing like kale,
collards, and turnip greens. They contain a lot of calcium.

One way of cooking greens is to steam them lightly.
They are ready to eat when they begin to sweat, or are
covered with a fine dew of moisture. They still retain their
green freshness and will be very slightly crunchy.

Cooking a big bunch of greens is a production and
can take as long as two hours, depending on how many
there are. Although they cook down, you may be left with
about two quarts of greens that you can enjoy all week long
if you do not eat a lot of them at one sitting. Greens cooked
in the way I am about to describe are also excellent in a
sandwich of pita bread.

In sesame oil or olive oil, in the bottom of a large
enamel stock pot or, if fewer greens, in a large dutch oven, I
saute two or three onions until they are dark brown. While
they are cooking on a medium-high flame and I am occa-

sionally stirring them, I am chopping greens (which I have washed!), First I split the leaf down the middle, including the stem. When the leaves are all split, I start chopping.

After cutting off the tip of the stems, I chop the stems including the lower portion of the leaf. I throw them in the pot with the onions as I cook, stirring them from time to time to see that all get cooked and don't stick to the bottom of the pot. Then I chop the middle portion of all the leaves, and put them in the pot as I chop them. I may have to add a little water (one quarter cup or less at a time) to keep them from sticking. Then I chop the tenderest portion: the top of the leaves, and throw them in the pot, stirring them in little by little.

When all greens are chopped and in the pot, I usually need to add liquid, so I add a bit of soy sauce to taste, but not to make the greens too salty. I continue to stir until all the greens are cooked, occasionally adding a little water or perhaps more soy sauce. They are irresistible eaten immediately, and welcome any time thereafter. You don't need fatback to make great greens!

Before the greens have finished cooking, I like to grind in vast amounts of black pepper. It enhances their smoky flavor. Leftover greens can be served with lemon juice, but I like them as they are. They are a lot of work but worth it.

When I was sick I was told to cook greens "waterless". In a thick iron saucepan (can be hard to come by these days) I laid chopped, freshly washed greens, put on the lid and turned the flame to medium high. After 5-10 minutes, when the greens were nearly cooked, I added a tablespoon of soy sauce, stirred the greens about, replaced the lid, and turned the flame high for about one minute. Delicious! And a lot easier than the above method. Other vegetables can be cooked in this way also. Please consult your nearest macrobiotic cookbook.

A sweet delight

If you crave sweets, boil together for about a half hour in the following: an onion, a carrot, two slices of butternut squash, and a quarter cabbage. Discard the vegetables (they will be mushy except perhaps for the squash) and allow the liquid to cool. Save it in the refrigerator and drink a little from time to time. But warm it before drinking. The natural way is to not stress our body with extremes of any kind, including temperatures.

Another sweet snack is to spread tahini (sesame butter) or olive oil with rice syrup, or just the rice syrup itself, on whole grain toast. I like fruit jam, but those which are sweetened with apple or pear juice, not with sugar (sucrose). Apple or pear butter is nice. But these treats are not for the seriously sick, not for right now.

Should you be sick or have cancer, it is best, for now, to eat nothing sweeter than an occasional small handful of (organic: preserved without sulfur) raisins. As time went by, I took to putting currants and pine nuts or almonds in my bulgar (cracked wheat) with onions, to make it a little more exotic.

A nice dish for winter is to cook chestnuts with rice: dried chestnuts (in Oriental groceries) with short or medium grain brown rice. This requires first soaking the chestnuts for 2 or more hours. It was almost a joke, among persons with cancer, that we were so sugar-deprived that we drank the sweet soak water from the chestnuts instead of cooking the rice in it.

Liquid refreshment

Very little water is pure these days. Bottled water from the supermarket may contain trace amounts of alcohol. It is better to filter your own if you do not have a reliable (tested) well. To drink and cook with heavily or even moderately chlorinated water can endanger your health.

The macrobiotic way of living naturally calls for eating and drinking small amounts. I once had lunch with a saint, who said to me: "Eat little; live long." In addition to water, the favored teas are those made from one kind of herb only (not blends). When I had cancer, I drank kukicha: tea made from the pan-roasted twigs of the tea plant. This tea is very rich in vitamin A, is alkalinizing, and has little if any caffeine. Sometimes I had dandelion root tea; sometimes tea made from water left from boiling pan-roasted rice or barley or even, when sickest, from boiling a piece of kombu.

While the above information might help a person to get started eating in a very simple way, the properties of each plant are so powerful and special that it is wise, if you are sick, to see a macrobiotic counsellor who has studied at the Kushi Institute and who understands how to balance the foods in relation to each person's physical condition.

By eating close to nature, we can recover the instinctive knowing of what foods we may need to eat at any particular time, to stay in balance or to recover our balance.

My only authority for offering the above recipes and comments about food comes from my fifth visit to Michio Kushi who this time told me, although I was not yet well, "Don't come back. You know how to cook." So there I was, on my own and taking full responsibility for my food as medicine, my medicine as food. It was a scary situation, but just what I needed in order to gain confidence to face a life without cancer..